Multicultural Aesthetics in Facial Plastic Surgery

Editor

J. REGAN THOMAS

FACIAL PLASTIC SURGERY CLINICS OF NORTH AMERICA

www.facialplastic.theclinics.com

Consulting Editor
J. REGAN THOMAS

August 2014 • Volume 22 • Number 3

ELSEVIER

1600 John F. Kennedy Boulevard • Suite 1800 • Philadelphia, Pennsylvania, 19103-2899

http://www.theclinics.com

FACIAL PLASTIC SURGERY CLINICS OF NORTH AMERICA Volume 22, Number 3
August 2014 ISSN 1064-7406, ISBN-13: 978-0-323-32011-5

Editor: Joanne Husovski
Developmental Editor: Susan Showalter

Facial Plastic Surgery Clinics of North America (ISSN 1064-7406) is published quarterly by Elsevier Inc., 360 Park Avenue South, New York, NY 10010-1710. Months of issue are February, May, August, and November. Business and Editorial Offices: 1600 John F. Kennedy Blvd., Suite 1800, Philadelphia, PA 19103-2899. Periodicals postage paid at New York, NY, and additional mailing offices. Subscription prices are $390.00 per year (US individuals), $525.00 per year (US institutions), $445.00 per year (Canadian individuals), $653.00 per year (Canadian institutions), $535.00 per year (foreign individuals), $653.00 per year (foreign institutions), $185.00 per year (US students), and $255.00 per year (foreign students). Foreign air speed delivery is included in all *Clinics* subscription prices. All prices are subject to change without notice. POSTMASTER: Send address changes to *Facial Plastic Surgery Clinics*, Elsevier Health Sciences Division, Subscription Customer Service, 3251 Riverport Lane, Maryland Heights, MO 63043. **Customer service: 1-800-654-2452 (US and Canada); 1-314-447-8871 (outside US and Canada); Fax: 314-447-8029; E-mail:journalscustomerservice-usa@elsevier.com (for print support); journalsonline support-usa@elsevier.com (for online support).**

Reprints. For copies of 100 or more of articles in this publication, please contact the Commercial Reprints Department, Elsevier Inc., 360 Park Avenue South, New York, NY 10010-1710. Tel.: 212-633-3874; Fax: 212-633-3820; E-mail: reprints@elsevier.com.

Facial Plastic Surgery Clinics of North America is covered in *MEDLINE/PubMed* (*Index Medicus*).

Contributors

CONSULTING EDITOR

J. REGAN THOMAS, MD
Mansueto Professor and Chairman,
Department of Otolaryngology-Head and Neck
Surgery, University of Illinois at Chicago,
Chicago, Illinois

EDITOR

J. REGAN THOMAS, MD
Mansueto Professor and Chairman,
Department of Otolaryngology-Head and Neck
Surgery, University of Illinois at Chicago,
Chicago, Illinois

AUTHORS

EDUARD M. ALFANTA, MD, MPH
Clinical and Research Fellow, Philippine
Academy of Facial Plastic and Reconstructive
Surgery, Pasig City, Philippines; Fellow,
Philippine Band of Mercy, Quezon City,
Philippines

FAZIL APAYDIN, MD
Professor, Department of Otolaryngology,
Ege University Medical Faculty, İzmir, Bornova,
Turkey

J. KEVIN BAILEY, MD
Associate Professor, Division of Trauma,
Critical Care and Burn, Wexner Medical
Center, The Ohio State University,
Columbus, Ohio

ANTHONY BARED, MD
Foundation for Hair Restoration, Miami,
Florida

JOSE BARRERA, MD, FACS
Associate Professor, Uniformed Services
University; Chairman, Department of
Otolaryngology; Chief of Facial Plastic and
Reconstructive Surgery, San Antonio Military
Medical Center, San Antonio, Texas

MARK J. BEEN, MD
Facial Plastic and Reconstructive Surgery
Fellow; Private Practice, Cincinnati, Ohio;
Private Practice, Edwards, Colorado

JENNINGS R. BOYETTE, MD
Assistant Professor, Department of
Otolaryngology/Head and Neck Surgery,
University of Arkansas for Medical Sciences,
Little Rock, Arkansas

ANTHONY BRISSETT, MD, FACS
Associate Professor, Director of Facial Plastic
and Reconstructive Surgery, Bobby R. Alford
Department of Otolaryngology–Head and Neck
Surgery, Baylor Facial Plastic Surgery Center,
Baylor College of Medicine, Houston, Texas

ROXANA COBO, MD
Coordinator, Service of Otolaryngology, Centro
Médico Imbanaco, Cali, Colombia

JEFFREY EPSTEIN, MD, FACS
Associate Voluntary Professor, Department
of Otolaryngology, University of Miami College
of Medicine; Foundation for Hair Restoration,
Miami, Florida; Foundation for Hair
Restoration, New York City, New York

DAVID B. HOM, MD
Professor and Director, Division of Facial
Plastic & Reconstructive Surgery, Department
of Otolaryngology-Head & Neck Surgery,
University of Cincinnati College of Medicine,
Cincinnati, Ohio

YONG JU JANG, MD, PhD
Professor, Department of Otolaryngology,
Asan Medical Center, University of Ulsan
College of Medicine, Seoul, Korea

GORANA KUKA, MD
Colic Hospital, Belgrade, Serbia

SAMUEL M. LAM, MD, FACS
Director, Willow Bend Wellness Center, Plano,
Texas

DEVINDER S. MANGAT, MD, FACS
Professor of Facial Plastic Surgery; Private
Practice, Cincinnati, Ohio; Private Practice,
Edwards, Colorado; Department of
Otolaryngology Head and Neck Surgery,
University of Cincinnati, Cincinnati, Ohio

RAMSEY F. MARKUS, MD, FAAD
Director of the Laser Center, Department
of Dermatology, Baylor College of Medicine,
Houston, Texas

DAVID NOLEN, MD
Fellow, Facial Plastic and Reconstructive
Surgery, UC Davis Medical Center,
Sacramento, California

AMY LI RICHTER, MD
Bobby R. Alford Department of
Otolaryngology–Head and Neck Surgery,
Baylor College of Medicine, Houston, Texas

JULIAN M. ROWE-JONES, FRCS (ORL)
Consultant Nasal Surgeon, Department of
Otorhinolaryngology – Head & Neck/Facial
Plastic Surgery, Royal Surrey County Hospital
NHS Trust; Consultant Surgeon & Director,
Private Practice, The Nose Clinic, Guildford,
Surrey, United Kingdom

FRED J. STUCKER, MD
Professor, Department of Otolaryngology/
Head and Neck Surgery, Louisiana State
University Health Sciences Center—
Shreveport, Shreveport, Louisiana

JONATHAN M. SYKES, MD
Professor and Director, Facial Plastic and
Reconstructive Surgery, UC Davis Medical
Center, Sacramento, California

J. REGAN THOMAS, MD
Mansueto Professor and Chairman,
Department of Otolaryngology-Head and
Neck Surgery, University of Illinois at Chicago,
Chicago, Illinois

MARTY O. VISSCHER, PhD
Director, Skin Sciences Program; Associate
Professor, Division of Plastic Surgery,
Department of Surgery, Cincinnati Children's
Hospital Medical Center, University of
Cincinnati College of Medicine, Cincinnati,
Ohio

DAVID M. WEEKS, MD
Clinical Instructor, Department of
Otolaryngology – Head and Neck Surgery,
University of Illinois, Chicago, Illinois

Contents

discusses approaches to surgical correction of common anatomic variations. In addition, common pitfalls are outlined.

 A video of a septal extension graft accompanies this article

Mestizo patients are the largest ethnic minority in the United States; the main facial plastic procedure they request is rhinoplasty. Mestizo noses are a challenge. It is common to find bulbous, undefined nasal tips sitting on a poorly structured osteo-cartilaginous framework. A structural approach is presented whereby support structures of the nose are strengthened and reinforced with structural grafts. A gradual approach to the nasal tip is presented whereby sutures and grafts are used to improve rotation and projection and create more definition. Cases showing long-term results are presented with discussion of the different surgical techniques used.

This article discusses in detail the cultural aesthetic issues that confront the surgeon interested in performing Asian blepharoplasty in terms of defining an aesthetic Asian ideal and the subject of natural and ethnic preservation of identity. The surgical methodology of how to perform a full-incision–based Asian blepharoplasty is outlined in a stepwise fashion along with the perioperative concerns (preoperative planning and counseling, nature of recovery, and complications and revision surgery).

Patients of different ethnicities have specific characteristics that are essential for hair transplant surgeons to understand so that aesthetic results can be achieved. In this article, the approaches of follicular unit extraction and follicular unit grafting or strip hair transplants for pattern hair loss are reviewed, along with the procedures of eyebrow and beard transplants and surgical hairline advancement/forehead reduction surgeries, within various ethnic groups.

The demand for facial rejuvenation and cosmetic procedures is rising among all ethnicities and skin types. The authors present a review of lasers and how to select a laser based on skin type and the treatment goals of laser resurfacing: skin laxity, dyschromia, hair removal, keloid, and hypertrophic scarring. In addition, they discuss preprocedural and postprocedural considerations, potential complications, and their management to maximize patient outcomes and minimize risk.

Facial resurfacing procedures are becoming increasingly popular. The percentage of non-Caucasian individuals seeking these treatments continues to rise. Patients with darker skin types (Fitzpatrick skin types IV–VI) face unique challenges for successful facial skin resurfacing. Common issues encountered by non-Caucasian patients include dyschromias, acne scars, photoaging, keloid and hypertrophic scars, benign cutaneous tumors, and hair-related disorders. This article discusses the most frequently used lasers and chemical peels used to address these problems.

Patients and clinicians use skin color attributes such as color uniformity, color distribution, and texture to infer physiologic health status. Normalization of skin color, surface texture, and height are important treatment goals in the treatment of scars. Skin color, structure, and response to trauma, vary with ethnicity. The incidence of hypertrophic and keloid scar formation is influenced by these inherent skin attributes. Skin type influences the response to various modalities including laser therapy and surgical intervention, and skin differences must be considered in treatment planning to achieve optimal results.

Aging of the face is inevitable and undeniable. This process includes a loss of skeletal support, soft tissue volume depletion, and a decrease in skin elasticity. The contribution of these 3 factors varies between individuals with noticeable hereditary influence. Characteristic ethnic features have been described in the literature, but as societies have changed, many of these ethnic variations have blended together. Facial cosmetic procedures must to be tailored to address these variations in anatomy, and consideration must be given to enhancing the facial skeleton, adequately lifting the soft tissues, and planning careful incisions to be closed under no tension.

FACIAL PLASTIC SURGERY CLINICS OF NORTH AMERICA

FORTHCOMING ISSUES

Pediatric Facial Reconstruction
Sherard S. Tatum, *Editor*

Rhinoplasty: Contemporary Innovations
Richard E. Davis, *Editor*

Midface Rejuvenation
Anthony P. Sclafani, *Editor*

RECENT ISSUES

May 2014
Neck Rejuvenation
Mark M. Hamilton and
Mark M. Beaty, *Editors*

February 2014
**Techniques in Facial Plastic Surgery:
Discussion and Debate part 2**
Fred G. Fedok and
Robert M. Kellman, *Editors*

November 2013
Complications in Facial Plastic Surgery
Richard L. Goode and Sam P. Most, *Editors*

August 2013
Hair Restoration
Raymond J. Konior and
Steven P. Gabel, *Editors*

RELATED INTEREST

Dermatologic Clinics, Volume 32, Issue 3, April 2014
African Skin and Hair Disorders
Nonhlanhla P. Khumalo, *Editor*

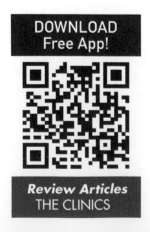

Preface
Multicultural Issues in Facial Plastic Surgery

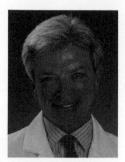

J. Regan Thomas, MD
Editor

As facial plastic surgery technology, techniques, and approaches continue to evolve, it is of key importance to recognize that our patients and their needs are evolving and changing as well. Changing concepts of beauty and desired appearance of the face and its anatomic structures are changing. The demographics of the world have evolved and thus the facial plastic surgery practice must adjust accordingly. The world and the patients encountered by the facial plastic surgeon are increasingly globalized. This is due to many factors, including population shifts and migration, cross-cultural interaction, racial identity, as well as racial and ethnic blending. This trend can no doubt be expected to continue with ongoing diversification of those demographics throughout the world. Indeed, as the world diversifies around us, impacting our facial plastic surgery patient encounters, our understanding of a variety of anatomic differences, ethnic and cultural goals, and global concepts of beauty must continue to become broader and more sophisticated.

This issue includes authors who are expert surgeons from a variety of ethnic, geographic, and cultural backgrounds. The reader will benefit from the approaches delineated in each topic based on the tremendous experience and expertise possessed by those individuals. Topics and procedures covered include rhinoplasty, blepharoplasty, facelift, skin resurfacing and skincare, hair replacement, and scar revision. Overall, the issue strives to educate the reader to a broader and more sophisticated approach in modern practice. I am honored to bring together this talented and diverse group of experts to develop this issue of *Facial Plastic Surgery Clinics of North America*.

J. Regan Thomas, MD
Department of Otolaryngology-Head and
Neck Surgery
University of Illinois at Chicago
Chicago, IL, USA

E-mail address:
thomasrj@uic.edu

Facial Plast Surg Clin N Am 22 (2014) ix
http://dx.doi.org/10.1016/j.fsc.2014.06.001
1064-7406/14/$ – see front matter © 2014 Published by Elsevier Inc.

Beauty in a Multicultural World

David M. Weeks, MD*, J. Regan Thomas, MD

KEYWORDS

- Multicultural appearances • Definitions of beauty • Facial appearance • Divine ratio
- Facial symmetry • Attractiveness

KEY POINTS

- Many ideals of beauty are stable, but surgical trends and techniques seem less enduring.
- Patients can rarely be characterized as fitting in a narrow mold with predictable surgical desires.
- Increased demand for cosmetic surgery has come from a more diverse, informed, and selective patient population from all walks of life.

INTRODUCTION

In today's world, beauty has a very important place. People are instantly judged as being outwardly attractive or not, and increased beauty confers remarkable advantages socially, reproductively, and professionally. Beauty crosses ethnic boundaries and has a huge cultural and economic impact.

The ancient Greek poet Sappho (seventh century BCE) stated What is beautiful is good. A century later, Plato postulated that what is good and true is beautiful.[1] Literature is filled with examples of villains being ugly and the ugly being evil. Meanwhile, the beautiful hero often swoops in to save the day. That being said, beauty has been a recognized entity for centuries yet we still struggle to define it. The irony is that most of us know it when we see it.

The face is a prime symbol and representation of the self. We carry photographs of the faces of our loved ones on our telephones or have them on our desks; our faces are displayed on our passport or driver's license to indicate who we are; it is the faces of criminals that adorn the news each night and the faces of famous persons on the covers of magazines. Our faces are the chief site for conveying our voluntary and involuntary emotional expressions.[2] Our faces largely define who we are and what kind of mood we are in.

Is facial beauty a simple or complex idea? Are there a set of ideals or measurements that aesthetically pleasing faces across all ethnicities have in common? Those are questions that provoke lively conversation and debate even among experts of facial analysis. Beauty was once considered to lie in the eyes of the beholder. This was a way of saying that beauty was subjective and ill-defined; a certain face may appear attractive to some people but unattractive to others. However, more recent studies have supported a more objective and well-defined concept of beauty. Certain concepts of facial beauty may indeed be timeless. Those concepts include symmetry, averageness, youth, and sexual dimorphism. Many studies have looked into the details of these characteristics.

The modern society is a truly globalized one and this has a definite impact on the perception of beauty. Interracial couples have increased, there is ubiquitous migration, and heightened economic mobility allows for a blurring of ethnic identity.[3] Mixed races and nationalities are the new norm, and this blending of traits often leads to

Department of Otolaryngology – Head and Neck Surgery, University of Illinois, 1855 West Taylor Street, MC 648, Room 2.42, Chicago, IL 60612, USA
* Corresponding author. Division of Facial Plastic and Reconstructive Surgery, Department of Otolaryngology – Head and Neck Surgery, University of Illinois, 1855 West Taylor Street, MC 648, Room 2.42, Chicago, IL 60612.
E-mail address: dmweeks4@hotmail.com

Facial Plast Surg Clin N Am 22 (2014) 337–341
http://dx.doi.org/10.1016/j.fsc.2014.04.005
1064-7406/14/$ – see front matter © 2014 Elsevier Inc. All rights reserved.

aesthetically unique and beautiful outcomes. Patients can rarely be characterized as fitting in a narrow mold with predictable surgical desires. People who identify with a certain ethnicity may want to erase, preserve, modify, or even enhance those specific inherent traits. Surgical goals must be tailored to the individual now more than ever.

Although many ideals of beauty are stable, surgical trends and techniques seem less enduring. Rhinoplasty has evolved into a far less destructive, less "operated on" appearance in the past decade. Blepharoplasty is trending toward fat preservation and redistribution. Few patients are looking for dramatic changes and most vehemently fear the surgical look. Surgical trends have often chased seemingly whimsical fads, whereas perhaps we should be more focused on the classical tenets of beauty.

Beauty has a critical role in mate selection, with more attractive persons being unconsciously perceived as being more fertile. It takes energy and natural resources for a body to create a beautiful exterior, and animals that are burdened with illness need to spend internal resources to fight off disease and cannot afford to devote energy to creating a beautiful, symmetric, or colorful exterior.[4] Attractive features confer an increased reproductive fitness, because sexually selected characteristics evolve much more quickly than naturally selected characteristics.[5] The beautiful are more likely to get better grades in school, to be hired for a job, and to receive higher salaries.[2] The drive to be beautiful is innate because nature stamps the more symmetric and youthful appearing as a beautiful individual, disease free, genetically fit, and fertile.[4] Beauty is a strong driving force in the world of nature and humanity alike.

PHI

The ancient Greeks believed true beauty was represented by a golden ratio, phi, of (a+b)/a = 1:1.61803399....[6,7] This has also been called the Divine Ratio because it is found throughout nature and is thought to represent perfect harmony. It is the ratio obtained when a line ABC is cut such that AB/AC = BC/AB. It has been used much in such well-known entities as Egyptian art and architecture and the Fibonacci sequence, and it is also found in basic geometric shapes, such as the pentagon and decagon. It is also found in the spiral of seashells, such as the nautilus; in the human mandible and its growth rate; in the spiral of DNA; and in the human figure and face.[8,9]

Phi has been studied extensively and some studies have found it to be inexact. Pallett and coworkers[10] found that individual attractiveness is optimized when the face's vertical distance between the eyes and the mouth is approximately 36% of its length, and the horizontal distance between the eyes is 46% of the face's width. This differed from the classic golden ratio of .38. He deemed his findings the "new" golden ratio and believed it to match those of an average face. Similarly, Schmid and coworkers[11] found that a face length to width in proportion less than the golden ratio are seen as attractive in female faces. Others have found phi to fit the female face more closely than the male face.[12] Furthermore, Pallett and coworkers[10] hypothesize that changing one's hairstyle may alter the perceived face length or face width, and their related length and width ratios, therefore affecting the perceived attractiveness of the face. Phi is a universal reference point for beauty, and it has certainly stood the test of time. However, its use does seem somewhat limited and it must be supplemented by additional mechanisms of facial evaluation.

SYMMETRY

The role of symmetry has been investigated as to its involvement in facial beauty. Most studies indicate that symmetric female and male faces are seen as more attractive than asymmetric ones. Some studies go so far as to say that there is a direct correlation with facial symmetry and attractiveness. This could be a result of symmetry alone, or it could be because symmetric faces are closer to the average than asymmetric ones.[13] Additionally, having a symmetric face seems to confer an advantage in sexual competition[14–17] because facial symmetry has been suggested to reflect a person's phenotypic and genetic condition.[18] It seems that an asymmetric face is not unattractive merely because it is asymmetric, but because the asymmetry implies moving away from the average, which in turn decreases reproductive fitness.

AVERAGENESS

Averageness and beauty initially seem to be mutually exclusive concepts. However, multiple people have studied this idea and a recurrent theme is that beauty and symmetry increase with increased averageness of facial features. Some people believe that facial averageness is the characteristic that contributes the most to facial attractiveness in women.[13] In 1979 Symons[19] performed a study where multiple single faces were artistically melded into a composite face. The composite face became increasingly closer to the average as the number of faces generating it rose. By increasing the number of faces it was also found that the composite face was increasingly more attractive.[19] This has been shown across multiple cultures and in other studies. Langlois and Roggman[20] created a composite face from many individual faces to test this concept and found that college students preferred the composite to any of the individual faces. The more faces that were used to construct the composite, the more attractive it was deemed.

Averageness is associated with a genetic and reproductive advantage. This can be explained by Darwinian theory, which suggests that evolutionary pressures operate against the extremes of the population.[21] Therefore, it can be postulated that averageness is attractive to potential mates because we innately appreciate that such mates represent genetic heterozygosity and have a greater probability of passing along our genes.[22]

The attractiveness of a female face depends on the averageness of most of its features but with deviation from the average of some local features.[13] Perrett and coworkers[23] used computer-generated digital imaging techniques to create a composite image of persons found most attractive and also to create a caricature of the more attractive composite to exaggerate the differences between it and the average composite by 50%. When tested with female faces, subjects preferred the more attractive composite to the average and the caricature to both. A different group of subjects, when tested with similarly constructed male faces, preferred the more attractive composite to the average, but there was no additional preference for the caricature. To examine cross-cultural differences the same procedure was followed with Japanese faces as judged by Japanese subjects, with similar findings. When composites of Japanese faces were shown to white subjects the results were also the same.[23] This study illustrated that facial beauty seems to be an objective and cross-cultural concept. Additionally, these studies show that deviation from the average on some individual characteristics can actually increase beauty and attractiveness.

YOUTHFULNESS AND NEOTENY

It seems obvious that youthful faces are deemed to be more attractive than older faces. Large eyes and small noses are considered attractive features, in part because it is believed that they represent youthful characteristics. Female faces digitally manipulated to have larger eyes were found more attractive than the original pictures with normal eyes and the ones manipulated to have smaller eyes.[24] This preference for neotenous features was found across a range of ethnic populations.[24–27] Neonatal features are thought to suggest desirable qualities of youthful vivaciousness, open-mindedness, and agreeableness.[13] As the female ages, her cheeks descend. Jowling occurs as the cheek fat pad falls over the jawline, causing the chin to become square-like and masculinized. The brows descend and the eyes become relatively smaller. The face deviates from the phi standard and attractiveness decreases. The mind interprets these changes as aging and of decreased fertility.

SEXUAL DIMORPHISM

Sexual dimorphism is defined as a phenotypic difference between males and females of the same species. For women in particular, a high estrogen-to-testosterone ratio in puberty results in fat deposits in the lips, upper cheek, breast, and hip; lengthening and narrowing of the facial bones; paler skin; and hairlessness. Multiple studies show these facial characteristics enhance the femininity and facial attractiveness of women thus increasing males' desire for females who possess these traits.[13,24,28,29] These hyperfeminine features include a thin jaw, small chin, large widely spaced eyes, small nose, high cheekbones, and plump lips. A preponderance of these estrogen-derived features would suggest a fertile host and reproductive advantage.[21]

Women typically prefer men with physical features suggestive of high testosterone levels: prominent chins, square jaws, deep-set eyes, thin lips, heavy brows, and abundant hair.[29] As women near ovulation they prefer more masculinized faces (thereby gaining the heritable genetic benefits). However, when women are unlikely to conceive, they prefer a more feminized face (possibly an indicator of more willingness to stick around and invest in offspring).[12]

ATTRACTIVENESS

Facial attractiveness has been associated with many positive qualities. Attractive people are consistently judged to be nicer, smarter, and healthier. Researchers have found that there is a consensus on rating attractiveness across sexual orientations, ethnic groups, and ages.[20,24–27] Additionally, studies have consistently shown that persons with mixed-ethnicity heritage are deemed to be more attractive than single-ethnicity persons.[30–32] It is hypothesized that this is related to increased genetic diversity and heterozygosity being internally recognized as a reproductive advantage.

Although males and females generally agree on attractiveness[23,33] there do seem to be significant gender differences. Women have been shown to be held to a more specific and rigid beauty standard than men. For men, it is easier to fall into the "average" category because it is a more inclusive, heterogenous, and less well-defined group. However, for women this is not the case. Professional female models are thinner than 98% of women[34] and images of women are far less likely to stray from the young, thin, and very attractive ideal than are images of men. This causes women to compare their body to a homogenous, unattainably high standard, so they chronically feel bad about their appearance.[35]

RHINOPLASTY

Rhinoplasty is one of the most common cosmetic procedures performed in the world today. Cosmetic rhinoplasty now transcends all age, gender, socioeconomic, and ethnic classifications. Its growing popularity is attributed to more surgeons, better surgical technique, more predictable outcomes, safer anesthesia, and the advent of digital photography and computer imaging software to explore various cosmetic changes.

There has been an evolution of the desired rhinoplasty outcome over the past 50 years. The 1950s nose had a glaring swooped bridge, upturned or rotated profile, and narrow tip. The heavily destructive excisional techniques creating these changes frequently led to late complications, such as pinched tip, retracted alar rims, or a saddled dorsum. By the 1990s, we saw an increase in grafting with the goals of conservation and preservation being franchised. Currently, noses with a straighter and natural-appearing profile with a fuller middle vault and slightly wider tip are preferred. Additionally, the preservation of distinguishing ethnic features of noses is at an all-time high. No longer do all patients want the classic northern European nose because there is no one universal shape that appeals equally to all patients.

Persons of Latin American, African, Asian, and white descent have noses characterized by certain osseocartilaginous features. The Latin American, or mesorrhine, nose typically has a low radix, less projection, and acute nasolabial angle. The African, or platyrrhine, nose has a flatter nose with a very low radix, small and wide nasal bones, less projection, and an acute nasolabial angle.[36] The Asian nose is also a platyrrhine nose notable for a low dorsum, small and weak lower lateral cartilages, retracted columella, thick alar lobules, poor tip definition, and thick sebaceous skin.[37]

The white, or leptorrhine, nose has a strong dorsum, high radix, big and strong nasal bones and upper lateral cartilages, big septal cartilage, defined tip, greater projection and rotation, and thin skin.[36]

Certain ethnicities tend to share similar rhinoplasty preferences, and patients frequently want to preserve their cultural identity despite undergoing surgery. Today more than ever, the successful rhinoplasty surgeon must be flexible and adaptable to multiple ethnicities and patients' diverse surgical desires.

CULTURAL CONSIDERATIONS

In addition to the aforementioned nasal anatomic differences, other parts of the face are equally unique from culture to culture. The Asian face is notable for a widened mandibular arch, prominent mandibular angle, convex mandibular body, parotid gland hyperplasia, excessive subcutaneous fat, hypertrophic masseter muscle, and foreshortened chin. These anatomic traits result in a broad lower facial skeleton and overall oval facial structure, especially in females.[38] East Asian eyelids are well-known for their absent supratarsal crease, prominent subcutaneous fat, thicker eyelid skin and orbicularis muscle, and conspicuous epicanthal fold. Latin Americans, Africans, and whites have their own inherent facial characteristics, each of which must also be carefully considered before any surgical procedure.

SUMMARY

Reality television, surgical documentaries, and plastic surgery–based television dramas have all ignited a flurry of cosmetic surgical activity, and the acceptance of cosmetic surgery is at an all-time high.[35] With this increased demand for cosmetic surgery has come a more diverse, informed, and selective patient population from all walks of life. Virtually no two patients have the same background or cosmetic objectives. However, the classic tenets of beauty including phi, symmetry, averageness, youthfulness, and sexual dimorphism can be applied to persons of all ethnicities to assist in objectifying the abstract concept. As the world around us diversifies, so too must our understanding of beauty and our attempt to surgically define beauty.

REFERENCES

1. Hoerber RG. Plato's greater hippias. Phronesis 1969;9(2):143–55.
2. Synnott A. The beauty mystique. Facial Plast Surg 2006;22(3):163–74.

3. Kridel RW. Ethnicity in facial plastic surgery. Facial Plast Surg 2010;26:61–2.

4. Dayan SH. What is beauty, and why do we care so much about it? Arch Facial Plast Surg 2011; 13(1):66–7.

5. Bashour M. History and current concepts in the analysis of facial attractiveness. Plast Reconstr Surg 2006;118(3):741–56.

6. Atalay B. Math and the Mona Lisa: the art and science of Leonardo da Vinci. New York: Harper Collins Publishers; 2006.

7. Prokopakis EP, Vlastos IM, Picavet V, et al. The golden ratio in facial symmetry. Rhinology 2013; 51(1):18–21.

8. Thompson DA. On growth and form. New York: Dover; 1992.

9. Cook TA. The curves of life. New York: Dover; 1978.

10. Pallett PM, Link S, Lee K. New "golden" ratios for facial beauty. Vision Res 2010;50:149–54.

11. Schmid K, Marx D, Samal A. Computation of a face attractiveness index based on neoclassical canons, symmetry, and golden ratios. Pattern Recogn 2008; 41:2710–7.

12. Bashour M. An objective system for measuring facial attractiveness. Plast Reconstr Surg 2006;118(3): 757–74.

13. Baudouin JY, Tiberghien G. Symmetry, average-ness, and feature size in the facial attractiveness of women. Acta Psychol (Amst) 2004;117:313–32.

14. Gangestad SW, Thornhill R, Yeo RA. Facial attrac-tiveness, developmental stability, and fluctuating asymmetry. Ethol Sociobiol 1994;15:73–85.

15. Grammer K, Thornhill R. Human facial attractiveness and sexual selection: the role of averageness and symmetry. J Comp Psychol 1994;108:233–42.

16. Mealey L, Bridgstock R, Townsend GC. Symmetry and perceived facial attractiveness: a monozygotic co-twin comparison. J Pers Soc Psychol 1999;76: 157–65.

17. Thornhill R, Gangestad SW. Human facial beauty: averageness, symmetry, and parasite resistance. Hum Nat 1993;4:237–69.

18. Wayneforth D. Fluctuating asymmetry and human male life-history traits in rural Belize. Proc Biol Sci 1998;265:1497–501.

19. Symons D. The evolution of human sexuality. New York: Oxford University Press; 1979.

20. Langlois JH, Roggman LA. Attractive faces are only average. Psychol Sci 1990;1:115–21.

21. Thornhill R, Gangestad SW. Facial attractiveness. Trends Cogn Sci 1999;3:452–60.

22. Penton-Voak IS, Perrett DI. Consistency and indi-vidual differences in facial attractiveness judgements: an evolutionary perspective. Soc Res (New York) 2000;67:219–44.

23. Perrett DI, May KA, Yoshikawa S. Facial shape and judgements of female attractiveness. Nature 1994; 368:239–42.

24. Cunningham MR, Roberts AR, Barbee AP, et al. "Their ideas of beauty are, on the whole, the same as ours": consistency and variability in the cross-cultural perception of female physical attractive-ness. J Pers Soc Psychol 1995;68:261–79.

25. Jones D, Hill K. Criteria of facial attractiveness in five populations. Hum Nat 1993;4:271–96.

26. Jones D. Sexual selection, physical attractiveness and facial neoteny: cross-cultural evidence and implications. Curr Anthropol 1995;36:723.

27. Jones D, editor. Physical attractiveness and the theory of sexual selection: results from five popula-tions, vol. 90. Ann Arbor (MI): University of Michigan; 1996.

28. Cunningham MR. Measuring the physical in physical attractiveness: quasi-experiments on the sociobio-logy of female facial beauty. J Pers Soc Psychol 1986;50:925–35.

29. Keating CF. Gender and the physiognomy of dominance and attractiveness. Soc Psychol Q 1985;48:61.

30. Little AC, Hockings KJ, Apicella CL, et al. Mixed-ethnicity face shape and attractiveness in humans. Perception 2012;41:1486–96.

31. Rhodes G, Lee K, Palermo R, et al. Attractiveness of own-race, other-race, and mixed-race faces. Perception 2005;34:319–40.

32. Lewis MB. Why are mixed-race people perceived as more attractive? Perception 2010;39:136–8.

33. Langlois JH, Kalakanis L, Rubenstein AJ, et al. Maxims or myths of beauty? A meta-analytic and theoretical review. Psychol Bull 2000;126:390–423.

34. National Eating Disorders Association. Statistics: eating disorders and their precursors. 2002. Available at: http://www.nationaleatingdisorders.org/press-rom/press-releases/2009-press-releases/national-eating-disorder-association-unveils-powerful-provocative-ad-campaign.

35. Buote VM, Wilson AE, Strahan EJ, et al. Setting the bar: divergent sociocultural norms for women's and men's ideal appearance in real-world contexts. Body Image 2011;8:322–34.

36. Cobo R. Ethnic considerations of the crooked nose. Facial Plast Surg 2011;27(5):467–82.

37. Toriumi DM, Pero CD. Asian rhinoplasty. Clin Plast Surg 2010;37:335–52.

38. Kwak ES. Asian cosmetic facial surgery. Facial Plast Surg 2010;26(2):102–9.

Facial Aesthetic Surgical Goals in Patients of Different Cultures

Julian M. Rowe-Jones, FRCS (ORL)[a,b,*]

KEYWORDS

- Rhinoplasty • Rejuvenation surgery • Facial aesthetic surgery • Patient selection • Culture
- Body image

KEY POINTS

- Compare the patient's aesthetic and psychosocial aspirations and expectations with the related values of the patient's cultural background, particularly referencing those of their family and close community.
- Greater acceptance of or demand for aesthetic surgery by a culture does not mean greater understanding of outcome or acceptance of an adverse outcome.
- Interpret the patient's behavior in the context of their cultural values; do not prejudge the patient or their relatives and friends, whether enthusiastic or concerned.
- Ensure the patient's values related to general standards of courtesy and care are understood, respected, and addressed.
- Be aware that indicators of a potentially unsatisfactory outcome are common to all cultures.

INTRODUCTION

The purpose of facial aesthetic surgery is to improve the patient's psychological well-being. The primary responsibility of the facial aesthetic surgeon therefore is to determine whether they can meet the expectations of their patient. Specifically, this means determining whether it is possible to achieve the physical change the patient wants. If it is possible, the surgeon must be confident that he or she has the personal experience to achieve such possible changes. Of equal importance is determining whether achieving the aesthetic changes expected will lead to fulfillment of the patient's psychological expectations. Having carefully determined the patient's physical and psychological expectations,

the surgeon must be sure the patient has understood the risks and accepted that their expectations, although achievable, may not be met, or that an adverse event may occur, making their appearance worse.

In determining psychological motivations and expectations, it is increasingly recognized that body image is the critical factor to consider when assessing patients seeking aesthetic surgery, rather than looking for traditional diagnoses of psychopathology.[1] That is not, however, to say that disorders such as depression or personality disorders should be dismissed because they may be co-conditions predicting a poor outcome. Body image is the mental picture individuals have of how they appear to others. This

Disclosure Statement: No Conflict of Interest.
[a] Department of Otorhinolaryngology – Head & Neck/Facial Plastic Surgery, Royal Surrey County Hospital NHS Trust, Egerton Road, Guildford, Surrey, GU2 7XX, UK; [b] Private Practice, The Nose Clinic, St Mary's House, Guildford, Surrey, GU1 3PY, UK
* Private Practice, The Nose Clinic, St Mary's House, Guildford, Surrey, GU1 3PY, UK.
E-mail address: jrj@thenoseclinic.co.uk

Facial Plast Surg Clin N Am 22 (2014) 343–348
http://dx.doi.org/10.1016/j.fsc.2014.04.003

image is judged in relation to what the individual considers is normal. Although most patients are not asking to look beautiful, they do want to achieve what they perceive is an aesthetic standard, which they consider to be normal and therefore not abnormal, unattractive, or deformed. The patient's set standard against which they judge themselves and perceive others are judging them will be influenced by culture. The cultures contributing to this aesthetic standard may be that of the patient's own background and in the era of global communication that of other societies too. The surgeon must understand which cultural influences the patient is subject to and what they are.

MOTIVATIONS FOR SURGERY

There may be differences in the motivations of those seeking restorative aesthetic surgery as opposed to transformative surgery such as rhinoplasty. The restorative patient may be seeking rejuvenation or correction of changes caused by trauma but may have been satisfied with their appearance previously. However, their acquired change in body image through injury or age will still have led them to think they no longer meet their perception of society's standard aesthetic and so are judged adversely; this will have resulted in low social confidence and loss of self-esteem. Different cultures and different social classes within the same culture may attach different values to facial appearance. The degree of a patient's lack of social confidence will be proportional to the culture they reference. Duelling scars were popular among upper-class Austrians and Germans involved in academic fencing at the start of the 20th century. Deviated noses are accepted as badges of masculine bravery among rugby players today—a sport traditionally associated with higher socioeconomic groups. In lower socioeconomic groups, such an appearance may be interpreted as a sign of nefarious, pugilistic activity.

The surgeon must further distinguish between internally motivated patients looking to improve confidence and esteem and who have a better chance of a positive outcome and externally motivated patients. The latter are expecting not only to change their bodies but also the success of their lives, often in the hope of pleasing others. The Asian or Middle Eastern patient may expect to achieve greater career success or to increase their chance of marriage if they westernize their appearance with blepharoplasty or rhinoplasty. Although their close cultural peers may hold this to be likely, in the context of their broader society,

this outcome is unlikely to be true.[2] The cultural frame referenced by the surgeon must therefore not be too narrow.

AESTHETICS AND BEAUTY

The facial aesthetic surgeon must also understand the patient's interpretation of normal to be able to assess whether the degree of their body image concerns matches their perception of normal. It is equally important to appreciate also what the patient's community and peer group consider standard. The patient will not only be judging themselves against a standard but will also be perceiving society's judgment of them. The perceived standards will be very significantly influenced by culture and further by varying social groups' tastes within a culture. The facial aesthetic surgeon must understand the value a society or social group attributes to appearance, also influenced by culture. It seems that beauty and youth are the apparent new indicators of social worth.[3] This view contrasts with cultures wherein age may be revered and elders are deferred to with respect. Such cultural values will influence a patient's body image and provide a context for their decision to consider aesthetic facial surgery. In cultures where beauty and youth are attributed a high social worth value, the definition of this social worth may be different. One culture's perceived wisdom may be that a certain appearance may lead to a greater chance of marriage, another to increased corporate career success. As a surgeon, therefore, one must understand that what might be a false expectation in one's own culture might not be in our patient's culture. However, it is important to explain to the patient that the perceived wisdom of a culture, often influenced by powerful marketing, may be wrong.

The facial aesthetic surgeon must also appreciate that a culture or society will judge an individual's desire to undergo aesthetic surgery differently. What may be considered a positive action to increase one's psychological well-being by one culture might be considered vanity or a lack of psychological strength and conviction by another. This concept will help us understand the patient and their body image and expectations in the context of their cultural norms. The facial aesthetic surgeon can then better advise on the validity of their judgments and better determine whether their psychosocial expectations can be met.

It is interesting in this context, however, to consider whether there are any universal normals that the facial aesthetic surgeon can refer to that are independent of cultural influence. Is there a universal concept of physical facial beauty with an associated normal range of attractive appearance around a universal standard? If there is, across races and culture, then it makes it easier for us to determine whether our patients' requests are based on expectation of achieving a normal or not. Research does suggest that appreciation of facial attractiveness is innate and present in infancy. Furthermore, cross-cultural investigations reveal similar standards of beauty across diverse cultures.[4] Measuring beauty has been performed for centuries and all facial aesthetic surgeons understand the importance of analysis, which implies comparison with a normal value. Normal values relate to averageness, and averageness and symmetry are associated with attraction. Jefferson[5] proposes that there are universal standards for facial beauty in both frontal and lateral profile views and that racially and ethnically diverse faces possess similar facial features that are deemed desirable and attractive. He refers to Marquardt's beauty mask used for facial soft tissue analysis that describes beauty and is independent of race.

Outstanding beauty may necessitate multiple facial features being average or magnification or diminution of at least one feature. Fashion will determine what is magnified or diminished and will change the context and relationship of facial features with age and race. The fashion and entertainment industry with the increasing power, presence, and influence of modern media and marketing, used to create demand, will manipulate facial features to create new representations of beauty. These representations may not be attainable. Different cultures may be exposed to the same media images but have different levels of public scrutiny, comment, and perspective. Some of our patients therefore will not understand that what is portrayed as an aspirational, aesthetic appearance is unattainable. The associated lifestyles and relationships, that is, the social worth portrayed with these appearances, may erroneously be interpreted as highly likely sequelae of aesthetic surgery too. The facial aesthetic surgeon must explain to the patient that these expectations cannot be met.

THE VALUE OF APPEARANCE

Over time, some segments of a society may adopt the values and worth given to an aesthetic appearance that is promoted by the media and these values may attain validity in some cultures but not others. The surgeon therefore in judging their patient's motivation for surgery must not be governed by their own aesthetic references but by those of their patient's culture. However, it must be considered that the association of a particular appearance with a high social worth value is likely to be short-lived because fashion changes quickly and probably only represents the views of a small part of a cultural group. These views might more appropriately be taken to represent a taste rather than a cultural value. Although it would be convenient and easier for patient selection to accept Kant's proposal of an aesthetic universality, later sociologic study has associated aesthetic preference, which might therefore be considered as taste, with education and social origin. Choosing a specific aesthetic appearance may therefore be an appropriate means of displaying social distinction and hierarchy. Making a financial aesthetic choice therefore may seem to be an appropriate attempt to redefine one's social status in one culture even if not in another, which may be why Asian patients in the Orient request more extreme westernization than Asian patients in the west. However, even if a culture purports to value such a distinction, this may not be true in reality. Cosmetic surgery in East Asia in terms of employment or earnings prospects has been shown to be a bad investment.[2] As a surgeon, one may understand a patient's motivation but must advise from a broader context.

If it is perceived by a society that having a Caucasian nose or Caucasian eyelids equates with greater attractiveness and social standing and therefore a greater chance of marriage, as some middle eastern patients have suggested, the facial aesthetic surgeon must be aware that, although this could be an issue for society, it does not mean that the individual patient is necessarily psychologically out of step. It has been suggested in South Korea that cosmetic facial surgery is very common in girls because they are encouraged by their society to strive for brilliance in both studies and appearance and to believe that if they look like pop stars they will be more successful.[6] The surgeon, though, must be sure that society will promote those that look like pop stars.

Western society tends to exhibit a bias against advancing age with older women regarded as less feminine and less employable in the visual media. The vigorous, successful corporate man may also be perceived as younger. The visual effects of aging may therefore come to be considered as a pathology that should be treated and aging "corrected." Consequently, more people will think they do not meet the aesthetic standard for their age. Their body image will change and they may think not only that they are being judged negatively but also that they are suffering economic disadvantage. As such, greater proportions of those societies may consider rejuvenating surgery acceptable, beneficial, and worth the risk. Other cultures, however, may hold religious beliefs that consider undergoing surgery to change one's appearance unacceptable. Members of a culture or community may value a physical trait that is considered typical and representative of their social group. The patient's desire for surgery reflects disparity in a community or culture's physical standard and a more global aesthetic standard that has influenced their body image. Wishing to change facial appearance in these cultures may not be supported and may not meet the patient's psychosocial expectations or may even result in adverse reaction if they remain in their community. The facial aesthetic surgeon knows that adequate physical and emotional family and community support after surgery improves the chance of patient satisfaction. A patient's motivation for surgery must therefore be judged in the context of and in comparison with the held beliefs and values of their family, culture, and community's opinion leaders.

COMMUNICATION AND INTERPRETATION

Understanding our patient's psychological motivations and goals is perhaps one of the most challenging aspects of patient selection for facial aesthetic surgery. It can be very difficult for a patient to articulate what psychological benefit specifically means to them in their everyday life. Different cultures may interpret the same words and phrases differently. Clear communication is vital in achieving a good relationship between a patient and their clinical team and increases the likelihood of a satisfactory outcome, meaning the surgeon must understand what different cultures value when determining trust and levels of care provision. McCurdy[7] draws attention to the perceptions and expectations of surgery that are particular to the Asian patient. He highlights the postoperative period as an area in which expectations and behavior may differ significantly from Caucasian patients.

ADVISING PATIENTS

It is not the prerogative of the aesthetic surgeon to impose their taste on a patient and to make value judgments on different cultures' tastes. However, it is important to point out to patients that the standard they are comparing themselves to is influenced by fashion, which changes and in fact

may be artificial and unattainable. This may be particularly true for younger patients, particularly those living in the Middle and Far East who may be more influenced by Western fashion and media pressure. The facial aesthetic surgeon must be aware too for younger patients that body image is more likely to change over time. The facial aesthetic surgeon should point out too that cultural values are not fixed and change as society reflects on its values and evolves. Lam[8] states that using Western aesthetic values to inform the outcome of Asian surgery should be discouraged. He counsels that the Westernization of the Asian face sought 20 years ago is inappropriate now. This approach would fail to take into account current cultural sensitivities that seek to avoid an unnatural or overtly foreign appearance (**Fig. 1**). It is interesting to propose that these cultural changes may reflect increasing sophistication and consequent changes in contemporary marketing to different demographics and newly wealthy populations. Ironically though, as different societies and cultures start to value their identities, globalization of media-driven aesthetics and homogenization of the gene pool may lead to greater convergence of opinion on universal standards of beauty. As a surgeon, one should also step outside the perspective of their own culture's dogmas surrounding beauty and see different concepts with fresh eyes. This globalization may also result in greater acceptance of cosmetic facial surgery across cultures. It may be easier for the facial aesthetic surgeon to evaluate their patients' body image concerns and expectations regardless of cultural background.

A good technical result from aesthetic facial surgery today is considered to be one that is natural and does not look "surgical," which generally means avoiding excess resection or augmentation. Normal contours must be maintained and balance must be achieved between individual nasal units and the face. Not only is the Westernization of 20 years ago inappropriate for Asian or black patients today, but so is the more extreme reduction rhinoplasty performed for Caucasian noses 20 to 30 years ago. The aspiration for natural facial aesthetics, whether for transformation or rejuvenation, seems to be cross-cultural, perhaps giving credence to the notion of a universality of what is beautiful and of what is normal. It may be true too that the drive for a more natural result is an attempt to make aesthetic surgery more acceptable to a wider proportion of society and to increase the market size. This finding must be borne in mind for all cultures to avoid trivializing surgical interventions and their risks.

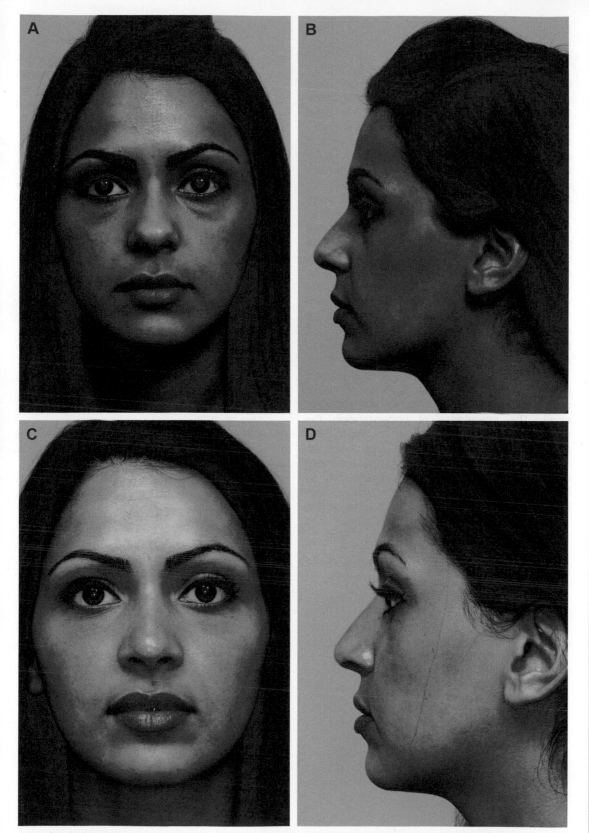

Fig. 1. (*A*, *B*) This patient requested tip refinement but wished to preserve her lateral profile dorsal convexity, which she thought was natural, balanced, attractive, and ethnically congruent. Using an open approach peri-domal, cephalic trims were performed, a columella strut inserted, and bilateral dome creation sutures and dome equalization sutures used. (*C*, *D*) Tip refinement and definition were achieved and tip position was maintained.

SUMMARY

Ultimately, the facial aesthetic surgeon must decide whether their patient's body image and the degree of concern associated with it is within the normal range. The surgeon must clearly understand whether the expected physical result and psychosocial improvements desired are within the normal range, which means understanding what is normal. Normal must be defined for appearance and for the value or social worth attributable to a normal appearance. These normals must be referenced to age. Culture and taste will influence values and aspirational standards and therefore by reverse extrapolation what is average or normal. In a global world, aesthetic values are probably finding common ground. It is valid for the surgeon to conclude that a wish for extreme change in any culture is cause for concern. It is valid for the surgeon to conclude that indicators of a poor outcome are common to all cultures.

Differences in fundamental aesthetic values, judgments, and aspirations may change slowly with time, but across cultures are probably small. The importance of understanding the values of individual cultures is to dispel false assumptions. Such knowledge also helps to determine whether the patient's values are those of a culture other than that of their family or community. Appreciating different values particularly helps the surgeon to be sensitive to factors that influence communication and comprehension on both sides. It also helps to demonstrate a more holistic understanding of the patients' needs at all stages of their journey, increasing the likelihood of a good doctor-patient relationship and outcome.

REFERENCES

1. Sarwer DB, Wadden TA, Pertschuk MJ, et al. The psychology of cosmetic surgery: a review and reconceptualisation. Clin Psychol Rev 1998;18:1–22.
2. Available at: http://www.asianplasticsurgeryguide.com/news10-2/081001_cosmetic-surgery-bad-investment.html. Accessed May 19, 2014.
3. Honigman R, Castle DJ. Aging and cosmetic enhancement. Clin Interv Aging 2006;1(12):115–9.
4. Alam N, Dover J. On beauty: evolutions, psychosocial considerations and surgical enhancement. Arch Dermatol 2001;137:795–807.
5. Jefferson Y. Facial beauty – establishing a universal standard. Int J Orthod Milwaukee 2004;15(1):9–22.
6. Available at: http://www.theatlantic.com/international/archive/2013/06/south-korean-high-schoolers-get-plastic-surgery-for-graduation/277255/. Accessed May 19, 2014.
7. McCurdy J. Preface. In: McCurdy J, Lam S, editors. Cosmetic surgery of the Asian face. 2nd edition. New York: Thieme; 2005. ix–x.
8. Lam S. Preface. In: McCurdy J, Lam S, editors. Cosmetic surgery of the Asian face. 2nd edition. New York: Thieme; 2005. xi–xii.

Rhinoplasty in the Middle Eastern Nose

Fazil Apaydin, MD

KEYWORDS

- Rhinoplasty • Middle Eastern nose • Thick skin • Dorsal hump

KEY POINTS

- In Middle Eastern noses, do not try to over-reduce nasal dorsum to make the nose smaller.
- Try to teach the behavior of thick skin to the patients.
- Support the tip structures.
- Try to keep the ethnic characteristics.

 A video of revision rhinoplasty on a Middle Eastern nose accompanies this article at http://www.facialplastic.theclinics.com/

INTRODUCTION

The Middle East is a region that roughly encompasses a majority of Western Asia and Egypt.[1] Twenty-eight ethnic groups live in 18 countries with Arabs, Turks, and Persians taking the lead. This is the area where world civilization started, and also this is the region for never-ending population changes throughout the history. Nevertheless, having the chance to visit, lecture, and operate in many of these countries, the author can say that there are many similarities in nose and face features.

In the literature written on the Middle Eastern nose, thick skin, dorsal hump, overprojected radix, wide upper two-thirds, nasal deviation, poorly defined and underprojected tip, weak lower lateral cartilages, acute nasolabial angle, and nostril tip asymmetries have all been reported to be seen with varying ratios.[2–6] In a photogrammetric study done in a Turkish population, crooked nose, obtuse nasofacial angle, and acute nasolabial angle were found to be the major problems for patients seeking rhinoplasty.[7] Similar results seem to be valid for Arabic noses as well.[8]

Traditional Turkish noses are usually big, with humps of varying degrees. The biggest humps are found in the Black Sea region of Turkey, where the longest nose on a living person recorded in the Guinness Book of World Records comes from.[9] In all the Middle Eastern countries, dorsal hump is almost invariably the primary reason for seeking rhinoplasty.

According to the author, the skin thickness of the nose increases in southern and eastern parts of the Middle East; this increase has also been reported in the literature.[3,10] Skin color also gets darker in a similar fashion. That is why triamcinolone injections are more popular in these countries. One of the major problems caused by skin thickness and darker skin is the increased visibility of external rhinoplasty incisions.[11,12]

TREATMENT GOALS AND PLANNED OUTCOMES

The challenge is that the use of a standard approach to the patients coming from different ethnic origins seems impossible. On the other hand, many of the problems for rhinoplasty patients in Middle Eastern countries show similarities, meaning a well-planned operative plan can be valid for most patients. The treatment goals for most patients can be summarized as follows:

1. Flat or slightly curved dorsal profile
2. Adequate tip projection and rotation

Disclosure: No disclosures.
Department of Otolaryngology, Ege University Medical Faculty, İzmir, Bornova 35100, Turkey
E-mail addresses: fazil.apaydin@ege.edu.tr; fazil.apaydin@gmail.com

Facial Plast Surg Clin N Am 22 (2014) 349–355
http://dx.doi.org/10.1016/j.fsc.2014.04.009

3. Better tip definition
4. Narrower and smaller nose
5. Better tip support
6. Middle vault reconstruction
7. Straight nasal septum

PREOPERATIVE PLANNING AND PREPARATION

One of the most important stages of rhinoplasty is to understand the goals of the patient, which necessitates a careful history taking. In the Middle East, the goals of patients may differ from country to country and from ethnic group to ethnic group. In some countries, the women are very eager to have very small noses and look more like a Caucasian. In the author's patients, the tendency is to have a nose that looks natural and functional.

When a patient is accepted to be operated by the author, 11 pictures are taken: frontal, laterals, obliques, basal, frontal smiling, lateral smiling, and 3 views by putting a ruler on 1 side of the head (frontal, lateral, basal). These pictures are transferred into Rhinobase, a computer program designed specifically for rhinoplasty patients, for aesthetic and photometric analysis.[13] After a thorough facial analysis in Rhinobase, the frontal, lateral and basal views (the ones including ruler) are transferred into Photoshop (Adobe Photoshop CS5 Version 12 [Adobe Systems Incorporated, San Jose, CA, USA]), where image processing is done with the patient in the consultation room. This stage is of utmost importance, because the patients express their requests; then the surgeon can simulate the desired shape and tell them how to reach these goals surgically and also the limitations in each individual case. Starting from the radix, the author usually tells his patients that he is usually reluctant to lower the radix while lowering the nasal dorsum, because it is too difficult to obtain a satisfactory result. While planning the dorsum, the author usually gives the female patients 2 options: a flat dorsum or a little curved one. Within the last decade, almost none of the patients the author saw have been seeking for overly done nasal dorsums. In the author's experience, it is not the same in all the countries in the Middle East. For example, in Iran many surgeons are still asked to make the noses very small with an overly reduced dorsum.

PROCEDURAL APPROACH

The author prefers to operate all his patients under general anesthesia. In 80% of the cases, an external approach is used. After the local anesthetic is applied, an inverted-V incision and marginal incisions are performed. The columellar flap is elevated by using sharp curved scissors, and the incision edges are cut perpendicular to the wound edges. Then the caudal end of the medial crura and the lateral crura are dissected. The middle third is dissected on a supraperichondrial plane and upper third in a subperiosteal plane. In recent years, the author generally has cut the perichondrium of the middle third in the midline and dissected it to both sides to skeletonize the medial aspect of the upper lateral cartilages. This layer can be of help to cover the middle vault just before closure. Usually the soft tissue in the interdomal, intercrural area and over the nasal spine is resected in order to minimize postoperative swelling and facilitate graft insertion. The depressor septi nasi is also usually cut at this stage, which can pull the footplates of the medial crura to destabilize the nasal tip. The caudal end of the nasal septum is exposed by using sharp dissection with a curved scissors. Half of the caudal segment is exposed, and then small tunnels under the cartilaginous dorsum are opened by using a Freer (Medtronic ENT, Jacksonville, FL, USA) elevator to facilitate the detachment of the upper lateral cartilages from the dorsal segment of the nasal septum. If there is a septal deviation or if septal cartilage is needed for grafts, the nasal septum is exposed bilaterally by keeping the 3 to 5 mm of mucoperichondrium attached to the cartilage at the level of the lower half of the dorsal segment. An L-strut of 12 to 15 mm is kept in place while harvesting the rest of the cartilaginous septum. If the bony septum is deviated, or long splinting spreader grafts are needed, then the bony septum is also harvested without breaking its attachment with the cartilage. In order to correct the difficult septal deviations, the rules of segmental reconstruction are applied.[14] The next step is to cut the upper lateral cartilage (ULC) from the nasal septum sharply by scissors or scalpel. In accordance with the preoperative plan, the amount of cartilaginous septum is resected by scalpel, and the bony part is removed by using Rubin osteotome. ULCs are turned in as spreader flaps when the amount of resection of the cartilaginous septum is more than 3 mm. Otherwise, spreader grafts are used to restore the middle vault or to correct deviations of the dorsum. The bony part is rasped to lower the upper third after the middle vault is reconstructed. At this stage, medial fading osteotomies are performed by 3 mm guided straight osteotome, followed by gentle rasping and irrigation.

Tip bulbosity and droopiness are 2 major problems encountered in the Middle Eastern nose. One of the author's favorite techniques to solve

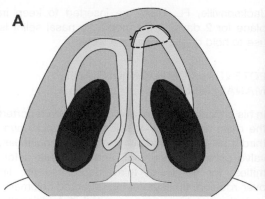
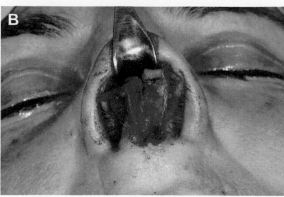

Fig. 1. The new domes technique is a very important tool to get rid of droopy tip. In the graphic depiction (*A*), it is seen that the suture steals 2-3 mm of cartilage from the lateral crus. In the intraoperative picture (*B*), the net gain in projection on the left side is clearly seen after putting the new dome suture.

both of these problems at once is the use of the new domes technique (lateral crural steal) (**Fig. 1**).[15,16] I think that this is an often neglected technique in the Middle East, and it is a versatile suture technique. In less droopy tips, domal sutures are used routinely. Depending on the width, shape, orientation, and resiliency of the lateral crura, many techniques can be employed. If the width of the lateral crura is more than 11 mm, modified lateral crural turn-in flaps are used. If used without detaching the scroll area, this technique helps to support both external and internal valves. Besides, they help to give a more favorable shape to lateral crura (**Fig. 2**).[17]

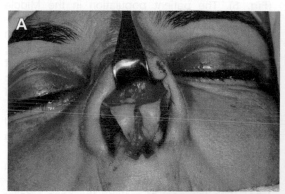
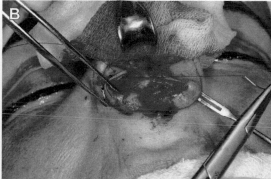
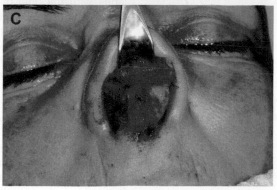

Fig. 2. Lateral crural turn-in flap is a very simple and effective technique to support and reshape the lateral crura by supporting external and internal valves at the same time. (*A*) The concave lateral crura are exposed by external approach. (*B*) Cephalic part of the lateral crus is turned in and sutured with the remaining caudal part by using matress sutures. (*C*) After the application of lateral crural turn-in flap on the right side, a more favorable shape of the lateral crus is obtained.

Cephalically oriented lateral crura are rarely encountered in the author's patients. According to the author, in patients with a droopy tip, the lateral crura may seem cephalically oriented, but when this condition is solved by increasing rotation and projection, the situation changes. Lateral crural strut grafts, alar battens, and alar rim grafts are all good options and quite often used by the author when additional support for the external valve is necessary, especially in revision cases.

After the domal suture and lateral crural interventions, the 2 domes are brought together by using transdomal suture.[18] Sometimes an additional dome equalization suture is also added. Septocolumellar suture is one of the workhorses of the author (**Fig. 3**). Starting from below, 2 mattress sutures are used where one of them usually brings 2 footplates closer. The power of this suture is its versatility to establish the desired rotation and projection in each case. Then a long floating columellar strut with a slightly curved shape is sutured between the medial crura (**Fig. 4**). As the last maneuver, lateral high-low-high osteotomies are done, and the profile is checked. If there are some depressions or irregularities, small thinned cartilage grafts or bruised cartilage grafts as camouflage can be used. These grafts are sometimes used as tip onlay grafts to give a better tip definition. The columellar incision is closed by 6-0 Vicryl Rapide (Ethicon, Somerville, NJ, USA) and the marginal incision with 5-0 Vicryl Rapide. After putting the quilting sutures in the nose, Doyle silicon splints (Medtronic ENT, Jacksonville, FL, USA) are inserted to keep in place for 2 days. A thermoplastic nasal splint is use to hold on the nose for a week.

POTENTIAL COMPLICATIONS AND MANAGEMENT

In his critical analysis of 500 cases, Foda reported the main reasons for revision in the upper two-thirds as dorsal saddling, dorsal irregularities, valve collapse, open roof, and pollybeak deformities; for the lower third, depressed tip, tip over-rotation, tip asymmetry, retracted columella, and alar notching were reported.[19] Additionally, the author sees recurrent septal deviations and crooked nose as well.

Over-reduction of the hump is a major problem encountered in Middle Eastern patients. Unfortunately, this is mainly because the surgeon's attempt to fulfill excessive demands of the patients. The patients are inclined to force the limits of resection and influence their surgeons to resect more. The author has observed some experienced surgeons form the Middle East trying to make a normal looking nose much smaller in accordance with the wishes of the patient (**Fig. 5**). The patient population in the Middle East is very keen on facial plastic surgery, especially with rhinoplasty, and colleagues in Tehran have named the city as the capitol of rhinoplasty, which might be probably true. Therefore, the first thing a surgeon from the Middle East should learn is how to balance the excessive demands of patients.

Problems related to the external and internal valve are 2 major problems, with patients seeking revision rhinoplasty in the author's experience. The main reasons are poorly handled septum and over-resection of the upper and lower cartilages with the goal of making the nose smaller (Video 1). In primary cases, the author has come up with the term, "minimal invasive functional rhinoplasty," in reduction rhinoplasties. In primary external rhinoplasty where the nasal septum is straight, the upper lateral cartilages are turned in as spreader flaps; the lateral crura are turned in as lateral crural turn-in flaps, and the resected cartilaginous septum from the hump is used as a columellar strut.

Recurrent crooked nose is another potential complication. The main reason for this complication is failure to correct severe septal deviations. In this kind of traumatic or severe deviation, the author follows the principles of segmental nasal reconstruction during the first surgery where reconstruction is much easier than revision cases.[14] In primary cases, one of the valuable graft

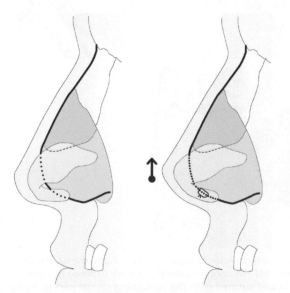

Fig. 3. Septocolumellar suture is a critical suture in defining both projection and rotation with 1 shot.

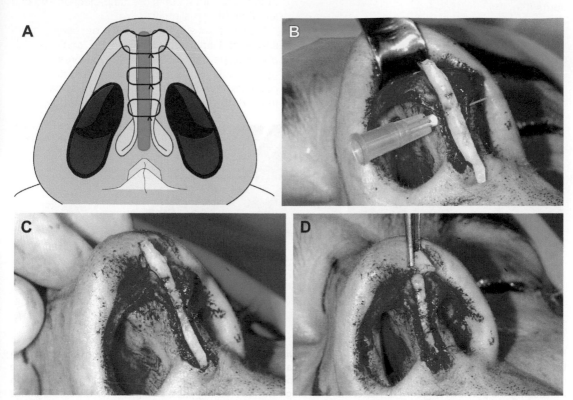

Fig. 4. The main reason why the author prefers long and curved columellar strut is the weak medial crura, which need to be supported throughout its entire length (*A*). The big strut is first fixed between the medial crura by a small needle (*B*); then it is positioned by multiple mattress 5-0 PDS sutures (*C*). The excess cartilage is then shaved to give the final shape to the strut (*D*).

sources is the bony septum. Straight pieces obtained from thin ethmoid or thinned vomer can be used for stenting the deviated dorsal and/or caudal segments of the cartilaginous septum (see Video 1).[20] In revision cases, conchal or costal cartilage can be needed for reconstruction.[14]

In the more southern countries such as Saudi Arabia and Egypt, the thick skin is really a big problem, which can easily cause the formation of pollybeak deformity. Besides whatever the surgeon does in terms of tip definition, it usually does not show itself because of the thick and oily skin. The experienced surgeons in the region usually know not to resect more; on the contrary, they resect less and support more, although the author has seen prominent surgeons still making aggressive resections. The author warns all his patients with thick skin that an ideal result is impossible and tries to lower the patient's expectations. Even though the patients seem to understand the situation, in fact they usually do not, and that is why the author is cautious in accepting to operate on patients with thick skin. The author tells these kinds of patients that the nose can be swollen for a couple of years.

Unfortunately the surgeons operating in the southern countries do not have the luxury to be picky, because a good many of their patients have thick skin. That is why they say that they apply triamcinolone on a routine basis in most of these cases.[21,22]

Anatomically, the skin is thicker at the radix, thinner on the rhinion, and thicker on the supratip. That is why it is classically reported to reduce less over the osseocartilaginous junction in order to get a straight profile.[23,24] However, in Middle Eastern noses, the author thinks that this is not the case, and a straight osseocartilaginous dorsum should be obtained in order to get a better profile in men and women (**Fig. 6**). The reason may be a slightly different response of the nasal soft tissue to resection of the bony cartilaginous hump than seen in European noses.

POSTOPERATIVE PERIOD

The patients are asked to come 2 days after surgery for splint removal (if there is any due to extensive septal work). The thermoplastic cast is kept in place for a week. An additional tape

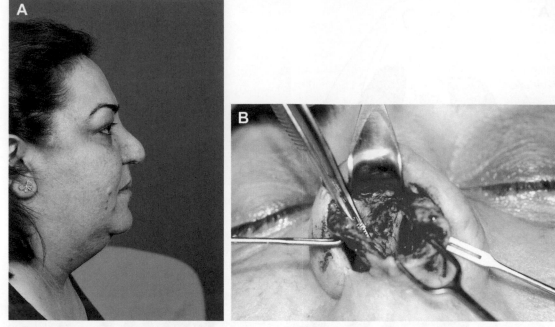

Fig. 5. A 52-year old female patient who has had 2 previous rhinoplasties and who still complains of a hump on the supratip region (*A*). During surgery, it was seen that too much cartilage has been taken from all over the dorsum, and the hump that the patient was complaining is simply scar tissue (*B*). The patient was successful in persuading the previous surgeons to resect more cartilage without leaving enough support for the cartilaginous framework.

application is done for another week. In crooked noses, patients are encouraged to apply mild massage to the nose from the deviated side. The author is not a fan of triamcinolone injections, unless there is a very heavy and thick skin. The patient is asked to come 6 weeks, 3 months, 6 months, 1 year and thereafter on a yearly basis for follow-up.

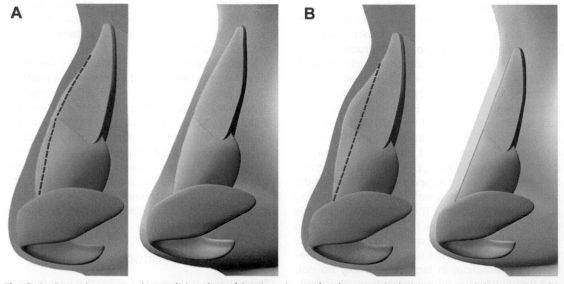

Fig. 6. In Caucasian noses, the traditional teaching is to leave the dorsum a little bit convex while resecting the hump in order to get a straight profile, because the skin is thinner over the key area (*A*). However, in Middle Eastern noses, this is not the case, and the dorsum should be straight during hump removal for a better looking profile (*B*).

SUMMARY

In Middle Eastern noses, each patient's concerns must be very thoroughly listened to, and the goals must be discussed with each patient. Segmental reconstruction of the nasal septum should be done in most cases. Over-reduction of the nasal dorsum should be avoided. Middle vault reconstruction by spreader flaps or grafts, and structural grafting techniques of the tip should be done in all cases. Thick skin can sometimes necessitate triamcinolone injections.

SUPPLEMENTARY DATA

Supplementary data related to this article can be found online at http://dx.doi.org/10.1016/j.fsc.2014.04.009.

REFERENCES

1. Available at: http://en.wikipedia.org/wiki/Middle_East. Accessed March 1, 2014.
2. Bizrah MB. Rhinoplasty for Middle Eastern patients. Facial Plast Surg Clin North Am 2002;10:381–96.
3. Rohrich RJ, Ghavami A. The Middle Eastern nose. In: Gunter JP, Rohrich RJ, Adams WP, editors. Dallas rhinoplasty: nasal surgery by the masters. 2nd edition. St Louis (MO): Quality Medical Publishing; 2007. p. 1139–65.
4. Rohrich RJ, Ghavami A. Rhinoplasty for Middle Eastern noses. Plast Reconstr Surg 2009;123:1343–54.
5. Daniel RK. Middle Eastern rhinoplasty in the United States: Part I. Primary rhinoplasty. Plast Reconstr Surg 2009;124:1630–9.
6. Azizzadeh B, Mashkevich G. Middle Eastern rhinoplasty. Facial Plast Surg Clin North Am 2010;18: 201–6.
7. Gode S, Tiris FS, Akyildiz S, et al. Photogrammetric analysis of soft tissue facial profile in Turkish rhinoplasty population. Aesthetic Plast Surg 2011;35: 1016–21.
8. Al-Qattan MM, Alsaeed AA, Al-Madani OK, et al. Anthropometry of the Saudi Arabian nose. J Craniofac Surg 2012;23:821–4.
9. Available at: http://www.guinnessworldrecords.com/longest-nose-on-a-living-person/. Accessed March 1, 2014.
10. Apaydin F. Rhinoplasty at the global crossroads. Arch Facial Plast Surg 2009;11:421–3.
11. Bafaqeeh SA, Al-Qattan MM. Open rhinoplasty: columellar scar analysis in an Arabian population. Plast Reconstr Surg 1998;102:1226–8.
12. Foda HM. External rhinoplasty for the Arabian nose: a columellar scar analysis. Aesthetic Plast Surg 2004;28:312–6.
13. Apaydin F, Akyildiz S, Hecht DA, et al. Rhinobase: a comprehensive database, facial analysis, and picture-archiving software for rhinoplasty. Arch Facial Plast Surg 2009;11:209–11.
14. Apaydin F. Segmental reconstruction for nasal septal deviation. Facial Plast Surg 2013;29:455–63.
15. Pedroza F. A 20-year review of the "new domes" technique for refining the drooping nasal tip. Arch Facial Plast Surg 2002;4:157–63.
16. Kridel RW, Konior RJ, Shumrick KA, et al. Advances in nasal tip surgery. The lateral crural steal. Arch Otolaryngol Head Neck Surg 1989;115: 1206–12.
17. Apaydin F. Lateral crural turn-in flap in functional rhinoplasty. Arch Facial Plast Surg 2012;14:93–6.
18. Tardy ME Jr, Patt BS, Walter MA. Transdomal suture refinement of the nasal tip: long-term outcomes. Facial Plast Surg 1993;9:275–84.
19. Foda HM. External rhinoplasty: a critical analysis of 500 cases. J Laryngol Otol 2003;117:473–7.
20. Apaydin F. Bone recycling in nasal septal reconstruction. Facial Plast Surg 2013;29:473–8.
21. Hanasono MM, Kridel RW, Pastorek NJ, et al. Correction of the soft tissue pollybeak using triamcinolone injection. Arch Facial Plast Surg 2002;4:26–30.
22. Guyuron B, DeLuca L, Lash R. Supratip deformity: a closer look. Plast Reconstr Surg 2000;105:1140–51.
23. Toriumi DM, Becker DO. Rhinoplasty dissection manual. Philadelphia: Lippincott; 1999.
24. Rohrich RJ, Muzaffar AR, Janis JE. Component dorsal hump reduction: the importance of maintaining dorsal aesthetic lines in rhinoplasty. Plast Reconstr Surg 2004;114:1298–308.

Rhinoplasty in the Asian Nose

 CrossMark

Yong Ju Jang, MD, PhD[a],*, Eduard M. Alfanta, MD, MPH[b,c]

KEYWORDS

- Asian rhinoplasty • Dorsal augmentation • ePTFE • Costal cartilage • Multilayer tip grafting
- Extracorporeal septoplasty • Short nose

KEY POINTS

- In augmentation rhinoplasty for Asian people, tip surgery using autologous cartilage followed by dorsal augmentation using alloplastic implant materials such as Gore-Tex (expanded polytetrafluoroethylene) or silicone is the most commonly performed procedure.
- Tip grafting procedures including shield grafting, multilayer tip grafting, and modified vertical dome division are mainstays in improving the Asian nasal tip.
- For severely deviated Asian noses, the senior author's modified extracorporeal septoplasty technique is useful before augmentation.
- A short-nose deformity is one of the typical problems in revision surgery for Asian people and requires the surgeon's best effort in correcting, using various maneuvers such as the use of extended spreader grafts and dorsal augmentation.
- Costal cartilage is an important graft material for Asian rhinoplasty; however, it is best reserved for primary surgery in thick-skinned individuals with poorly developed noses and complicated revisions.

ANATOMIC CHARACTERISTICS OF THE ASIAN NOSE

The tip of the Asian nose, particularly the east Asian or oriental nose, is usually low, and the lower lateral cartilages are small and weak. The nasal bones are flat and thick, resulting in a low radix. The average nasal length/nasal tip projection/dorsal height/radix height ratio of the nose in white people has been shown to be 2:1:1:0.75 (**Fig. 1**A).[1] However, in the senior author's study, young Koreans had a nasal length/nasal tip projection/dorsal height/radix height ratio of 2:0.97:0.61:0.28 (see **Fig. 1**B).[2] This finding supports the popularity of augmentation rhinoplasty to correct a low-profile nose among Asian people. Regarding the septum, the septal cartilage of some Asian people is thin and small. In a study

of the senior author's patients having external rhinoplasty, intraoperative measurement of the harvested septal cartilage was performed with preservation of L struts 10 mm wide. The mean caudal length of the harvested septal cartilage was 15.1 mm, and the mean dorsal length was 18.2 mm. Therefore, the size and the quantity of harvestable septal cartilage may be inadequate for complex rhinoplasty procedures, increasing the need of harvesting grafts from other sites.[3] Typical Asian noses tend to have thicker skin than noses of white people, with abundant subcutaneous soft tissue. In the senior author's research using computed tomography (CT) scans of the nose of Koreans, the mean nasal skin thickness was 3.3 mm at the nasion, 2.4 mm at the rhinion, 2.9 mm for the nasal tip, and 2.3 mm for the columella (**Fig. 2**). In this study, the thick skin at the

Disclosures: None.
a Department of Otolaryngology, Asan Medical Center, University of Ulsan College of Medicine, 88, Olympic-ro 43-gil, Songpa-gu, Seoul 138-736, Korea; b Philippine Academy of Facial Plastic and Reconstructive Surgery, Philippine Society of Otolaryngology – Head and Neck Surgery, San Miguel Avenue, Ortigas, Pasig City 1605, Philippines; c Philippine Band of Mercy, 22 East Avenue, Diliman, Quezon City 1100, Philippines
* Corresponding author.
E-mail address: jangyj@amc.seoul.kr

facialplastic.theclinics.com

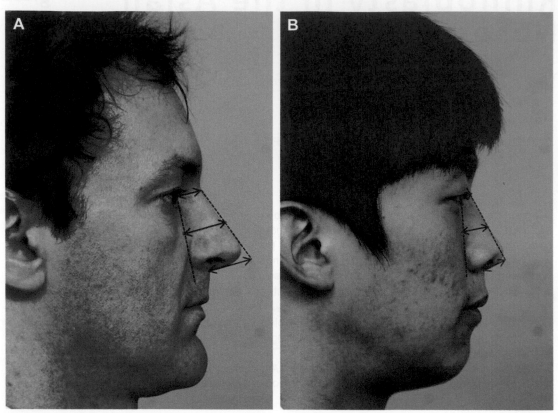

Fig. 1. (A) The average nasal length/nasal tip projection/dorsal height/radix height ratio of the nose in white people has been shown to be 2:1:1:0.75. (B) The average nasal length/nasal tip projection/dorsal height/radix height ratio of Korean noses has been shown to be 2:0.97:0.61:0.28.

nasal tip and columella was associated with poorer surgical outcomes, suggesting that regional skin thickness is an important prognostic factor for tip surgery success.[4]

AUGMENTATION RHINOPLASTY

The purpose of this procedure is the cosmetic improvement of typical low-profile noses without deviation, saddle or hump deformities, or a short-nose deformity.

Dorsal Augmentation

Dorsal augmentation is the most commonly performed procedure in Asian rhinoplasty. It is also critically important not only in simple cosmetic rhinoplasty but in all types of rhinoplasties in order to

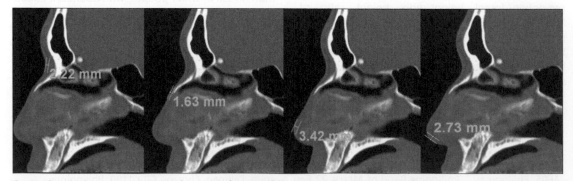

Fig. 2. Skin thickness was measured in several areas of the nose using CT scans. In this patient, the nasal skin thickness is 2.22 mm at the nasion, 1.63 mm at the rhinion, 3.42 at the nasal tip, and 2.73 mm at the columella. For Koreans, the mean nasal skin thickness was 3.3 mm at the nasion, 2.4 mm at the rhinion, 2.9 mm for the nasal tip, and 2.3 mm for the columella.

achieve aesthetic perfection. Unlike the rhinoplasty for white people, in Asian rhinoplasty, alloplastic implants still play an important role because of the differing anatomic characteristics of Asian noses, such as thick skin and poorly developed cartilaginous framework. There is no single ideal implant or graft for dorsal augmentation. Every material has its own merits and drawbacks.[5] Aesthetic perfection of the nose is determined by the height and shape of the nasal dorsum seen from the side and front, with its harmonious alignment with the nasal tip. The dorsal implant should be designed with the appropriate width, and the thickness of the patient's skin must be taken into consideration. In patients with thin skin, it is preferable to use soft implants such as expanded polytetrafluoroethylene (ePTFE) rather than silicone. In patients with thick skin, a more solid material such as silicone, reinforced ePTFE, or costal cartilage can be used without causing significant problems. In the senior author's experience, it is easier to get favorable aesthetic outcomes of dorsal augmentation when alloplastic implants are used, compared with the use of biological implants including autologous and homologous cartilage and fascia. Long-term follow-up of patients having rhinoplasty shows that aesthetic complications are more frequent in biological implants. These complications included visibility of the dorsal cartilage implant, warping, absorption, or deformation. Infections immediately following surgery are more common in biological implants, whereas delayed inflammations and infections are more common in alloplastic implants and if not treated adequately, can cause serious deformities.

Alloplastic implants
ePTFE and silicone are the most widely used alloplastic implants in Asian rhinoplasty (**Fig. 3**). ePTFE implants have microscopic pores that induce the surrounding tissue to grow into them, thus having the advantages of increased stability and lower incidence of capsule formation. In addition, the risk of extrusion is lower with ePTFE than with silicone. The soft texture of ePTFE reduces patient discomfort, and implant visibility through the skin is less common than with silicone implants.[6] ePTFE is available in different thicknesses. If a surgeon uses a sheet-type ePTFE implant of 1-mm to 2-mm thickness, multiple sheets should be stacked to get a sufficient increase in dorsal height. The advantage of using sheet implants is that augmentation levels can be adjusted for each region easily, even for patients with focal prominence or depression in the dorsum (**Fig. 4**). When using ePTFE, sufficient beveling of the

sheet's margins is essential, especially for sheets of more than 2-mm thickness. If not beveled correctly, the implant's margins can be felt through the skin after surgery. One notable disadvantage of ePTFE is that it decreases in volume after insertion.[7] In addition, it is more difficult to remove an ePTFE implant from the nasal dorsum than a silicone implant. Delayed inflammation is serious complication in the use of this material. It has been reported that the infection rate in primary surgery is 1.3%, whereas in secondary surgery it is 4.3% to 5.4%.[5]

Prefabricated silicone implants are the most popular material in dorsal augmentation for Asian noses. Because of its stable chemical structure, silicone has several advantages, including its low tissue reaction and ease of handling. Moreover, the availability of ready-made products makes implantation convenient, and the relative hardness of silicone makes it suitable for fashioning the desired nasal shape for Asian people with a moderately thick to thick skin.[8] Placement of an I-shaped implant at the nasal dorsum with tip plasty using autologous material (septal or conchal cartilage) is the preferred surgical method. When inserting silicone implants, the caudal end of the silicone implant should not be in direct contact with the tip skin. The caudal end of the implant is usually located in the space between anterior septal angle and alar cartilages, connecting the nasal dorsum with the nasal tip. Placement of stacked tip onlay grafts on the dome area, which is in direct contact with the tip skin, is frequently performed with silicone implantation (**Fig. 5**). Revision rhinoplasty after silicone implantation may be needed for implant deviation, floating, displacement, extrusion, impending extrusion, infection, and contraction of skin resulting in a short-nose deformity.

Autologous cartilage
Autologous materials are advantageous for dorsal augmentation of the nose because these implants are well tolerated and carry the least risk of infection. However, there is the issue of donor site morbidity. In addition, the aesthetic performance of these materials is generally worse than alloplastic implants, at least with respect to dorsal augmentation. Common autologous tissues used for dorsal augmentation include septal cartilage, conchal cartilage, costal cartilage, fascia, and dermofat.

Because it is easy to harvest and shape the septal cartilage, septal cartilage can be used to moderately elevate the nasal dorsum, to camouflage a partial concavity on the dorsum, and for nasal tip surgery. However, the use of septal

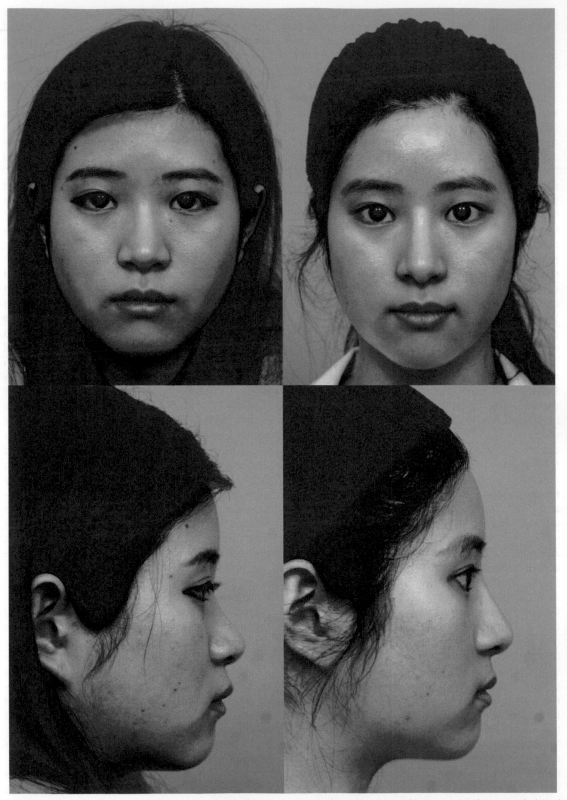

Fig. 3. A patient showing typical aesthetic changes after septal extension grafting, tip grafting, and dorsal augmentation using ePTFE. Before surgery (*left*), and 9 months after surgery (*right*).

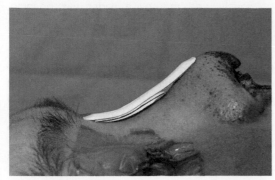

Fig. 4. Stacked ePTFE sheets tailored to conform to the nasal dorsum. The posterior surface of the implant can be carved to go over a focal prominence.

cartilage for dorsal augmentation is impractical in 1-piece dorsal augmentation of the noses of Asian people. First, it is difficult to obtain a long enough piece of cartilage (3–4 cm) for dorsal augmentation because the septal cartilage harvested is small.[3]

Second, using cartilage for cosmetic dorsal augmentation is less aesthetically pleasing compared with alloplastic implants because it is difficult to carve the cartilage as smoothly as alloplastic implants.

Conchal cartilage, unlike septal cartilage, has an intrinsic curvature that complicates its routine use in dorsal augmentation. In addition, the conchal cartilage is frequently too small to yield a cartilage piece suitable for 1-piece dorsal augmentation. A method avoid this problem is the use of diced conchal cartilage wrapped with fascia, and this has gained wide acceptance as an ideal dorsal augmentation technique.[9] However, conchal cartilage is preferred in tip surgery, but it is considered to be less suitable as dorsal augmentation material.

Although costal cartilage is difficult to harvest and is associated with serious donor site morbidities such as pneumothorax, as well as the problem of implant warping, it is the most useful

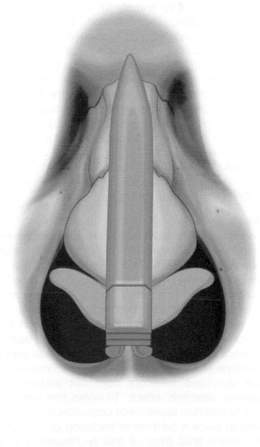

Fig. 5. Stacked tip onlay grafts on the dome area placed with silicone implantation to prevent the silicone implant from making contact with the nasal tip skin. Lateral view (*left*), and frontal view (*right*).

autologous cartilage for thick-skinned primary cases, which require substantial augmentation, or in patients who have experienced complications with alloplastic implants (**Figs. 6** and **7**).

Most rhinoplasty surgeons have difficulty using this cartilage at the nasal dorsum to form an aesthetically pleasing nose. This difficulty results in a high rate of aesthetic failure. In the senior author's experience, overall complication and revision rates of rhinoplasty using autologous costal cartilage are much higher than for rhinoplasty using other implant materials. Warping, graft visibility, and unnatural-looking noses are common complications of dorsal augmentation using costal cartilage.[10]

Surgery of the Nasal Tip

Asian noses reveal considerable diversity in the shape of the nasal tip. In the senior author's experience, tip suture techniques are not very useful in most Asian patients seeking greater projection and better definition, especially in patients who have thick nasal skin and weak alar cartilages. Thus, tip grafting procedures are the most common method of tip surgery for improving tip projection, rotation, and definition. They are also effective for improving tip support. As graft material, septal cartilage is preferred, but, when there is an insufficient amount or if the cartilage is thin and weak, conchal cartilage is the next best choice. In patients with extremely thick skin, use of costal cartilage as tip grafting material is a useful surgical option. The intrinsic shape of the alar cartilages in Asian patients usually manifests as an underprojected nasal tip with rounded contours. To make a fundamental change in this unfavorable tip shape, clinicians sometimes need to place multiple cartilage grafts on the tip.

Shield grafting

This is one of the most commonly used maneuvers to enhance tip projection and definition in Asian people.[11] This technique is usually effective in lengthening the infratip lobular segment, thereby enhancing tip projection. When executing this technique, if the shield graft is long, in addition to an increase in tip projection, an increase in the overall length of the columella is expected. Sometimes, a 1-layer shield graft made with weak septal cartilage easily bends cephalically after closure of the skin, and therefore does not achieve the desired aesthetic effect. To solve this problem and to maintain appropriate projection, it is necessary to place a buttress or backstop graft behind the shield graft (**Figs. 8** and **9**). Placement of a shield graft using conchal cartilage is another option, with the concavity of the cartilage facing caudally, acting like a spring to resist cephalic bending.

Multilayer cartilaginous tip grafting technique

Because of the diverse anatomic features of alar cartilage contours, placement of only 1 shield graft is insufficient to achieve the desired projection and definition in many cases. To overcome the limitations of conventional tip grafting techniques, the senior author uses a multilayer tip grafting technique in patients who have thick skin with bulbous and underprojected tips.[12] In multilayer tip grafting, the first cartilaginous shield graft layer is placed covering the caudal aspect of the middle to medial crura. Further graft layers are then placed on the caudal part of the first layer. The more caudal layer is placed so that its leading edge becomes higher than the existing dome and the layer(s) beneath it. The numbers of graft layers applied depend on how much projection is needed. As in a shield graft, a buttress or backstop graft is required in many cases (**Fig. 10**). The multilayer cartilaginous tip grafting technique maintains the advantages of shield-shaped tip grafts, which help in improving nasal tip projection and definition (**Fig. 11**), as well as enabling the surgeon to overcome issues relating to thick skin. This technique is versatile, so clinicians can easily adjust the height and vector of tip projection, and is particularly useful in lengthening the nose. The complications of this technique include transient tip erythema, infection, graft contour visibility, delayed-onset skin erythema, nostril deformity, and overprojection.[12]

Modified vertical dome division technique

Vertical dome division may be particularly useful for Asian patients with thick tip skin and well-developed lower lateral cartilages. The senior author has found that it is often difficult to gain the desired nasal tip refinement using vertical dome division alone, and so has devised a modification of vertical dome division.[13] In this modified vertical dome division technique, the incisions are made on both domes, borrowing a lot of cartilage from the caudal margin so that the lateral view of the medialized cartilages has a triangular projection in the anterocaudal direction. The vestibular skin is preserved through wide undermining along the medial and lateral crural surfaces. A cartilage strip, shaped like a columellar strut, is then placed between both limbs of the divided dome and is sewn together with the medialized domal portion of the lower lateral cartilages. A shield graft is then placed just in front of the newly created cartilage-strut complex. The leading edge of the shield graft is adjusted according to the desired

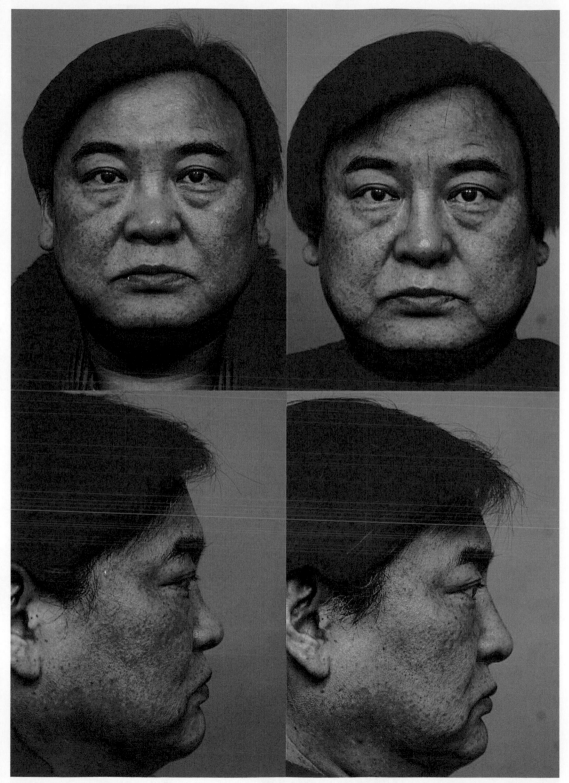

Fig. 6. A patient with thick nasal skin who underwent dorsal augmentation using costal cartilage. Before surgery (*left*), and 8 months after surgery (*right*).

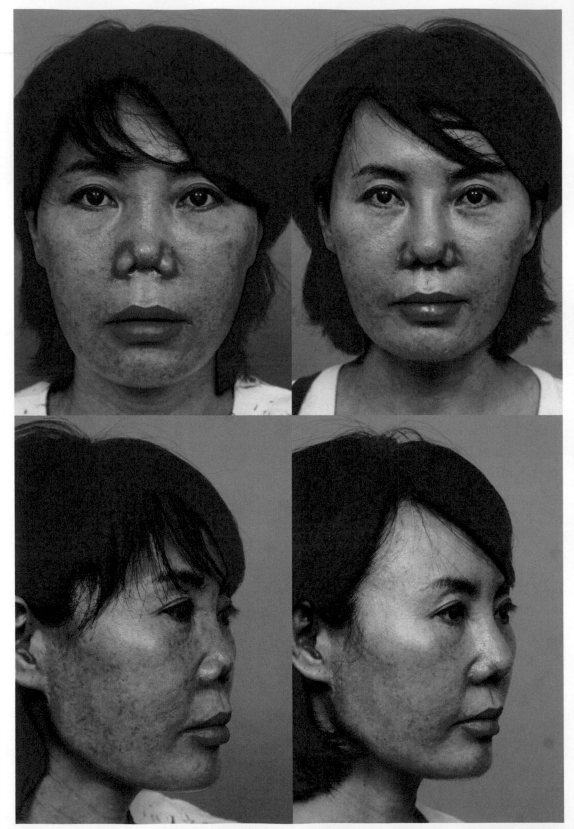

Fig. 7. Severe nasal distortion caused by silicone-related complications. Multiple grafts were placed, including dorsal augmentation using costal cartilage. Before surgery (*left*), and 3 months after surgery (*right*).

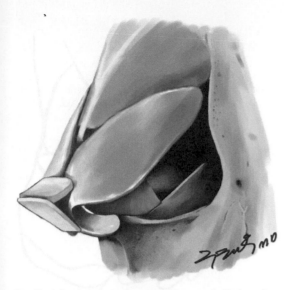

Fig. 8. A backstop graft preventing cephalic bending of a shield graft.

height of the new tip (**Fig. 12**). This modified vertical dome division technique is designed for patients with thick tip skin and strong, well-developed lower lateral cartilages (**Fig. 13**). Complications of this technique include excessive narrowing of the tip and tip asymmetry.

Tip onlay grafting

Tip onlay grafting is a procedure that places one or several layers of horizontally oriented grafts at the dome of the tip. It can be performed on a patient with proper tip support to increase tip projection, or to camouflage a tip irregularity.[14] Well-performed tip onlay grafting in combination with dorsal augmentation can produce a slight concavity in the nasal profile, which is favored by many Asian women (**Fig. 14**). If several layers of onlay grafts are positioned at the tip without any special manipulation of the lower lateral cartilages, even though the tip projection may be improved to some extent when viewed laterally, the infratip

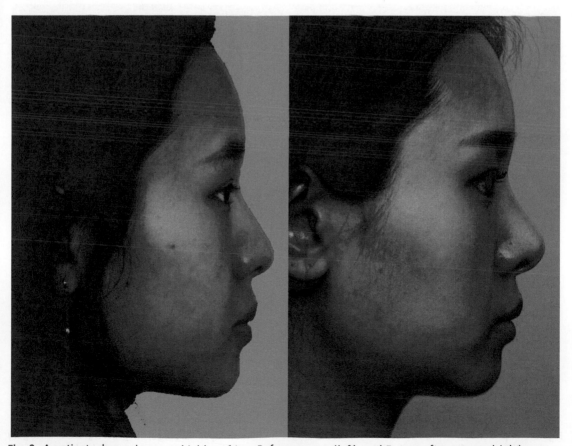

Fig. 9. A patient who underwent shield grafting. Before surgery (*left*), and 5 years after surgery (*right*).

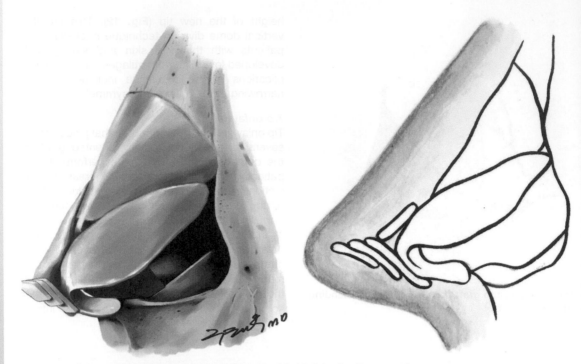

Fig. 10. Multilayer tip grafting without (*left*) and with (*right*) a backstop graft.

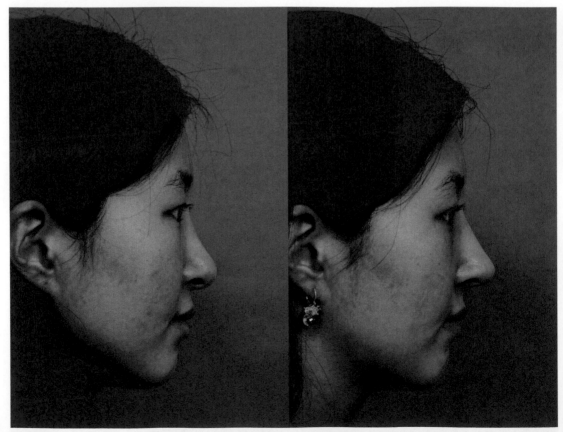

Fig. 11. A patient showing favorable aesthetic changes after multilayer cartilage tip grafting. Before surgery (*left*), and 2 years after surgery (*right*).

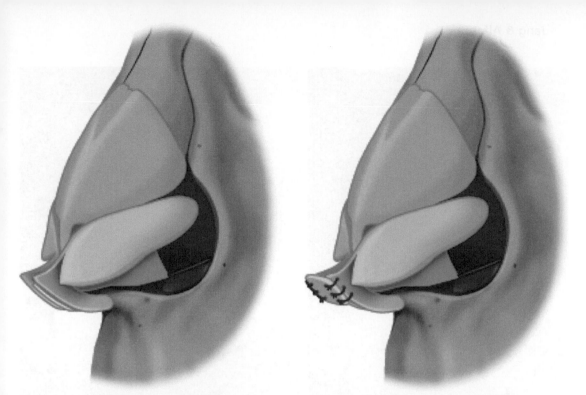

Fig. 12. Modified vertical dome division technique by the senior author. A triangular projection is created after medialization of the cut caudal cartilages. A cartilage strip is seen between both limbs of the divided dome, acting like a strut (*left*). A shield graft is then placed just in front of the newly created cartilage-strut complex (*right*). The leading edge of the shield graft is adjusted according to the desired tip height.

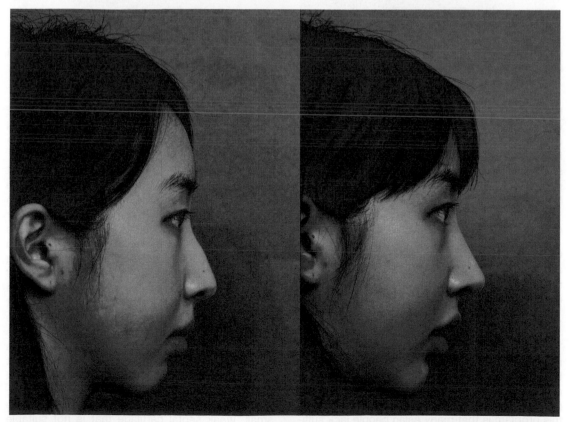

Fig. 13. A patient showing improved tip projection as a result of the modified vertical dome division technique. Before surgery (*left*), and 14 months after surgery (*right*).

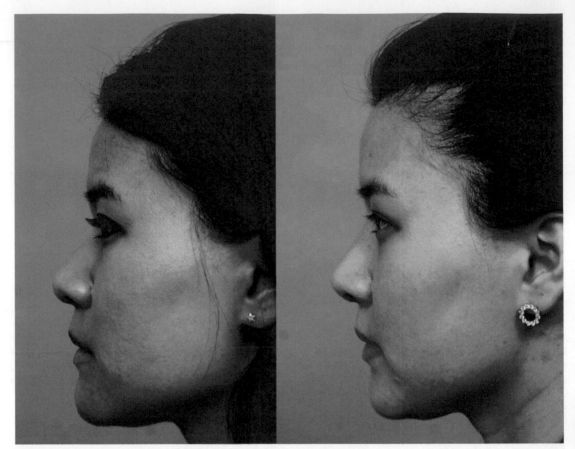

Fig. 14. Well-performed tip onlay grafting with dorsal augmentation can produce a subtle concavity in the nasal profile, which is favored by many Asian women. Before surgery (*left*), and 8 months after surgery (*right*).

lobule area can become excessively long when viewed basally, giving an unnatural appearance. Graft visibility can also be a common complication. In order to prevent this, the width of the graft should be almost equal to the width of the domal portion of the tip, and the graft margins should be properly beveled.

CORRECTION OF DEFORMED NOSES

Correction of Asian noses with deformities, such as deviation, dorsal convexity, saddle, and short-nose deformities, is another important element in rhinoplasty for Asian people.

The Deviated Nose

The surgical principles applicable to the management of the bony vault, middle vault, and lower third of the nose in white people are also applicable to the correction of deviated noses in Asian people. However, the issue in the management of this problem is that many Asian people lack sufficient septal cartilage for reconstructing the septal framework, tip surgery, and dorsal augmentation. The surgeon frequently must harvest additional cartilage to achieve complete correction of the deviated nose.

Correction of the nasal septum is the most important procedure, but is a difficult procedure in deviated nose surgery. A deviated septum can be corrected either using an in situ technique or extracorporeal septoplasty. In situ corrections involve degloving the septal cartilage and then making an L strut, which is straightened using various techniques and is left unresected. Typical in situ techniques include spreader grafting, batten grafting,[15] and cutting and suture of the L strut (**Fig. 15**).[16] The septal bone harvested during the septoplasty procedure is a useful material as batten grafting for the caudal or dorsal portions of the L strut (**Fig. 16**). Active use of this bony graft can reduce the need for harvesting additional cartilage, both in primary and revision rhinoplasties for Asian people, who frequently have small, weak septal cartilage that is not suitable for structural grafting.[17]

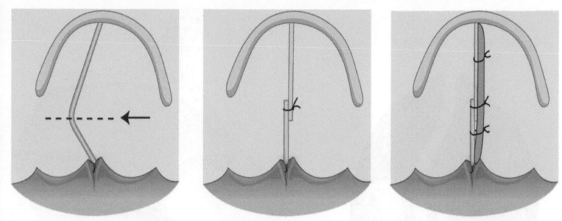

Fig. 15. Cutting and suture technique in the correction of the caudal L strut. Before correction (*left*), after cutting and suture technique correction (*center*), and after placement of a batten graft for additional support (*right*).

If the deviation of the nasal septum is too severe to be corrected with in situ techniques, extracorporeal septoplasty can be performed. This method involves removing nearly all of the nasal septum, and reimplanting it into position after reshaping it extracorporeally. The senior author prefers to perform his modification of the extracorporeal septoplasty technique.[18] In this modification, the osseocartilaginous skeleton is exposed through an external rhinoplasty approach. The septal cartilage is removed except for the remaining few millimeters of the dorsal strip at the keystone area. A straight and strong new L strut is then formed extracorporeally. The dorsal aspect of the new L strut is fashioned into a Y shape by suturing a cartilage strip to the existing L strut. The preserved cartilage tail at the keystone area is slotted in the fork of the arms of the Y-shaped cartilage and then sutured. Caudal septum stability is obtained by suturing the newly shaped septal cartilage to the soft tissue around the anterior nasal spine to create an inverted Y (**Fig. 17**).

If necessary, septal bone[18] or conchal cartilage can be harvested to be used as spreader grafts or batten grafts for better support. If the anterior nasal spine is deviated toward one side, the new septum should be sutured to the soft tissue of the contralateral side. This modified extracorporeal septoplasty is useful in treating severely deformed noses (**Fig. 18**). This technique obviates additional tip grafting because the height of tip can easily be altered by adjusting the caudal height of the extracorporeally designed septal cartilage.

Among the various different types of deviated noses, the linear deviation is the most difficult to treat.[19] Before beginning surgical treatment, the surgeon has to check carefully for facial asymmetry, which considerably limits a successful surgical

outcome. Many Asian patients desiring deviated nose correction also want an increased dorsal height after surgery. Dorsal augmentation can cover the irregularities created after the different surgical maneuvers. Thus, dorsal augmentation should be regarded as an important part in the correction of deviated Asian noses (**Fig. 19**).

Convex Dorsum of Asian Patients

Asian noses are generally smaller and less prominent than the noses of white people. The prevalence of a hump nose among Asian people is therefore less than in white people, but many Asian patients have hump noses. On examination of a patient, a typical hump or a humplike deformity can be identified. Therefore, it is desirable to define the deformities as a convex nasal dorsum. Convex nasal dorsum of Asian noses can be classified into 3 types: a generalized hump, an isolated

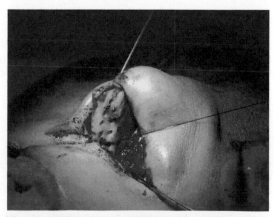

Fig. 16. Septal bone harvested during septoplasty used as batten grafting for reinforcement of the L strut.

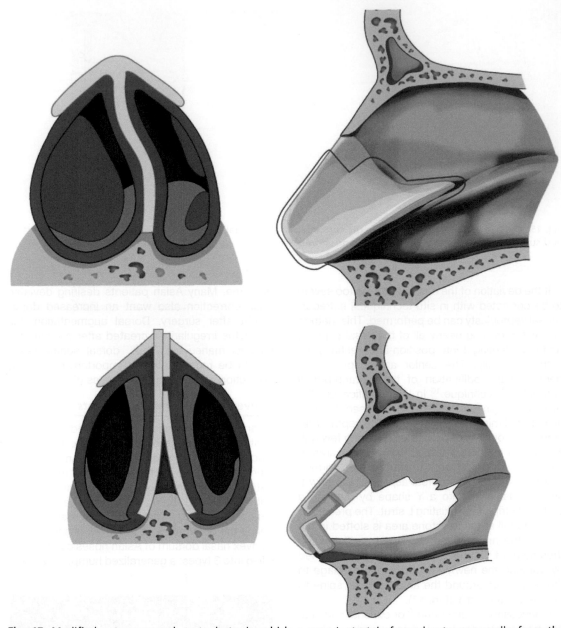

Fig. 17. Modified extracorporeal septoplasty, in which a new L strut is formed extracorporeally from the harvested septal cartilage. Precorrection axial view (*top left*), the portion of septal cartilage to be resected (*top right*), postcorrection axial view (*bottom left*), and the newly assembled L strut reimplanted (*bottom right*).

hump, or a relative hump with a low tip.[20] A generalized hump represents the typical hump deformity commonly seen in white populations, in which the curvature of the hump begins from the bony vault and extends to the cartilaginous dorsum in a gentle curve. An isolated hump represents an abrupt protrusion of a small hump in a triangular or round shape on the dorsal line. The hump is

short, with most of it located around the rhinion. A relative hump with a low tip is seen in patients in whom the nasal dorsum is not very high but the nasal tip is severely underprojected, giving a false impression of a nasal dorsal hump (**Fig. 20**).

In most cases of convex dorsum in Asian people, other than hump removal, tip augmentation and radix augmentation are important procedures

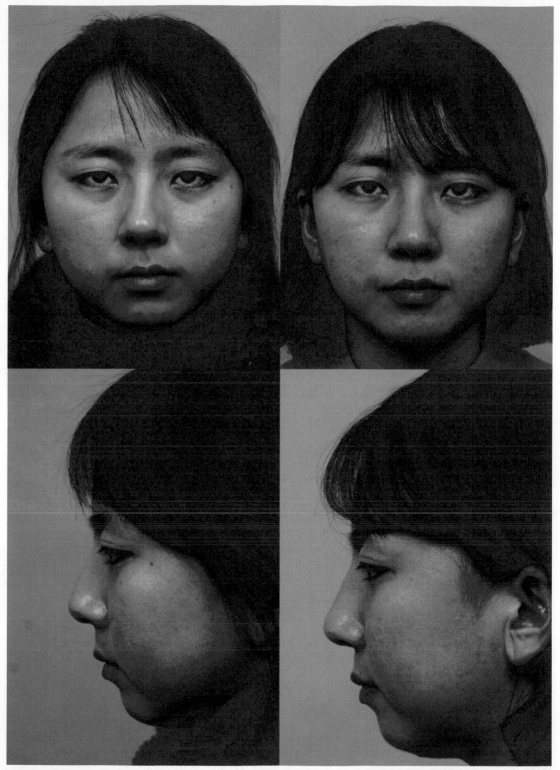

Fig. 18. Severe deviation of the nose corrected by extracorporeal septoplasty, osteotomy, and tip onlay grafting. Before surgery (*left*), and 1 year after surgery (*right*).

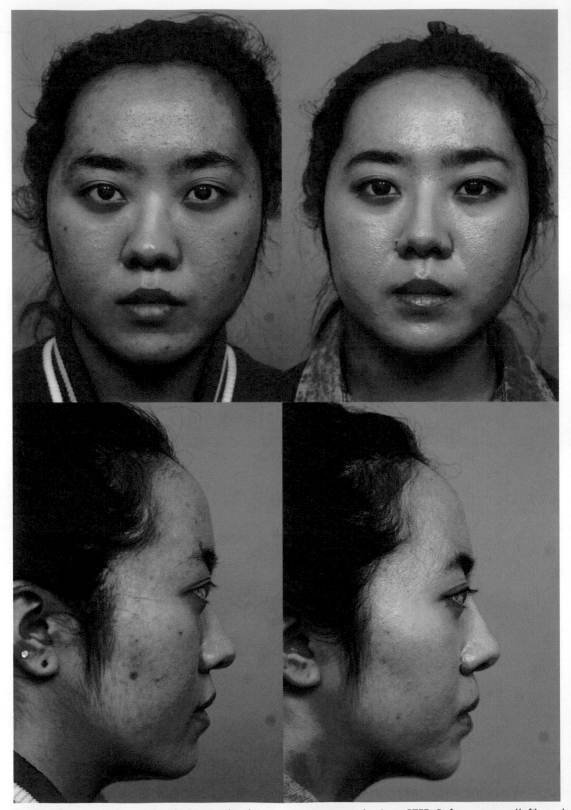

Fig. 19. After correction of the deviation, the dorsum was augmented using ePTFE. Before surgery (*left*), and 1 year after surgery (*right*).

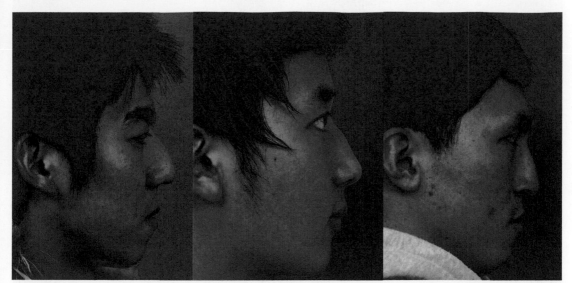

Fig. 20. Classification of convex dorsum according to the senior author. Generalized hump (*left*), isolated hump (*center*), and relative hump with a low tip (*right*).

for the successful management of hump noses (**Fig. 21**).[20] Because most Asian people lack appropriate tip projection, during the correction of the convex dorsum, the desired height of the tip should be set first, followed by the determination of the degree of hump reduction and augmentation of the radix and supratip according to the new tip height. For example, in a patient with an underprojected tip, if considerable improvement in tip height is desired, the surgeon does not need to reduce the hump, but instead should augment the supratip dorsum and radix, preserving the hump (**Fig. 22**). Thus the correction of a dorsal hump in Asian patients is closer to redistribution surgery than to simple reduction.

Short-nose Deformity

A short nose is one of the most difficult deformities to correct, and it requires the use of a multitude of challenging surgical techniques for adequate correction. A short nose most commonly develops as a sequela of nasal surgery, especially after dorsal augmentation with silicone or fascia.[21] In addition, overly aggressive rhinoplasty maneuvers that include extensive septal cartilage work are more likely to result in a short nose.

Successful correction of this deformity can be obtained by extending the internal framework of the nose and the external soft tissue envelope. In lengthening the nasal skeleton, an extended spreader graft using costal cartilage, multilayer tip grafting, and lateral crural strut grafting are important techniques.

A short nose is frequently accompanied by overrotation of the tip. The septal extension graft, particularly the extended spreader graft, is effective for lengthening short noses and counterrotating (derotating) the nasal tip. Various forms of septal extension grafts are defined, and the choice should be determined by the status of the native septal cartilage and the amount of available cartilage grafts. Sufficient lengthening of the nose can be more easily achieved by using a strong extended spreader graft made from costal cartilage. It is placed on both sides of the septum at a position that is 3 to 10 mm more caudal than the anterior septal angle. When the remaining L strut is thin and weak, the dorsal as well as caudal struts should be reinforced by strong and thick costal cartilage. Several methods are described in septal extension grafting (**Fig. 23**). Placement of the caudal graft in an end-to-end manner with the caudal septum sandwiched by the two extended spreader grafts is one useful technique. Placement of a batten graft on one side of the caudal strut and an extended spreader graft (extending more caudally) on the other side of the dorsal strut is another useful method.[22]

The nose appears shorter when the dorsum looks concave. Thus, the nasal dorsum must be augmented by an implant or graft. However, sufficient augmentation is often difficult to achieve because of the limited ability to stretch the skin-soft tissue envelope adequately in revision rhinoplasty, especially in silicone-implanted noses, in which the nasal skin is severely thickened, contacted, injured, or has lost its normal elasticity.

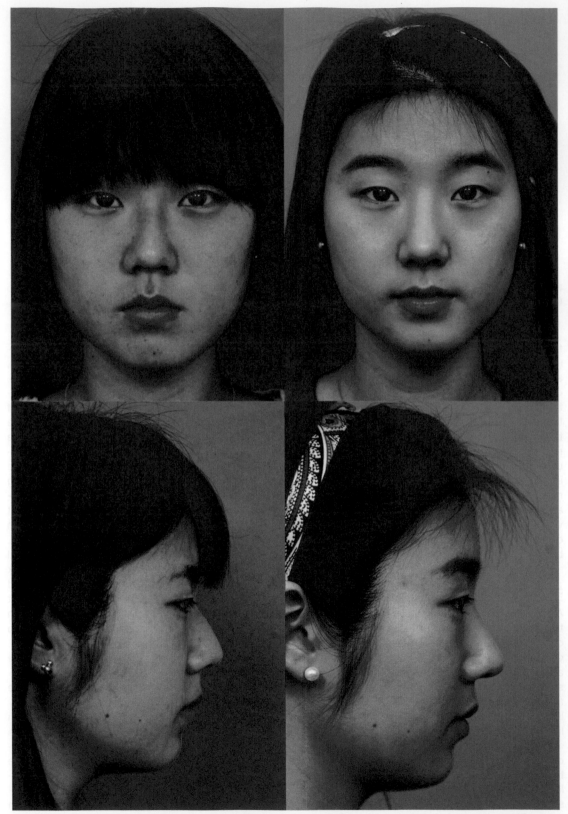

Fig. 21. A patient showing good results after hump reduction, spreader grafting, caudal batten grafting, and multi-layer tip grafting. The radix was augmented using fascia. Before surgery (*left*), and 2 years after surgery (*right*).

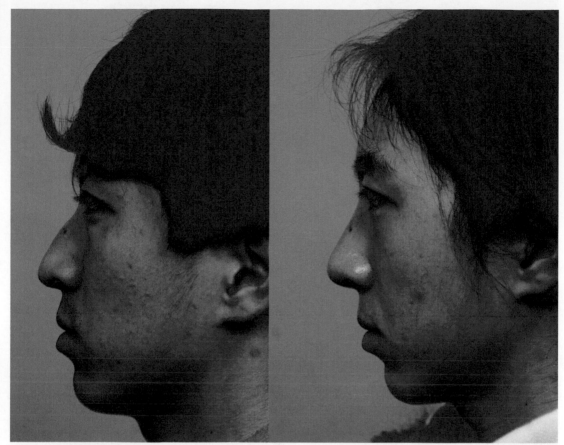

Fig. 22. A straight dorsal line was achieved by tip and radix augmentation without hump removal. Before surgery (*left*), and 1 year after surgery (*right*).

Therefore, lengthening of the nasal framework and dorsal augmentation should be performed within the range of the tension-free closure of the columellar incision. Because many patients have short noses resulting from the complications of silicone, removal of the silicone and insertion of another implant material is necessary, but, in these situations, there are limited options in selecting proper material. For this purpose, the senior author prefers to use costal cartilage, autologous or processed fascia lata combined with cartilage, as the dorsal implant material. ePTFE can also be used if the patient does not have signs of severe infection (**Fig. 24**).

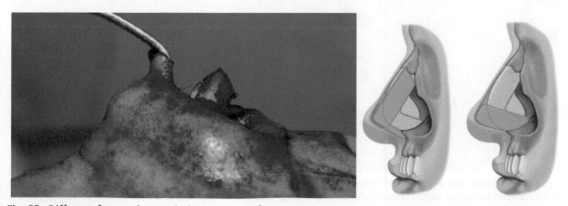

Fig. 23. Different forms of extended spreader grafts.

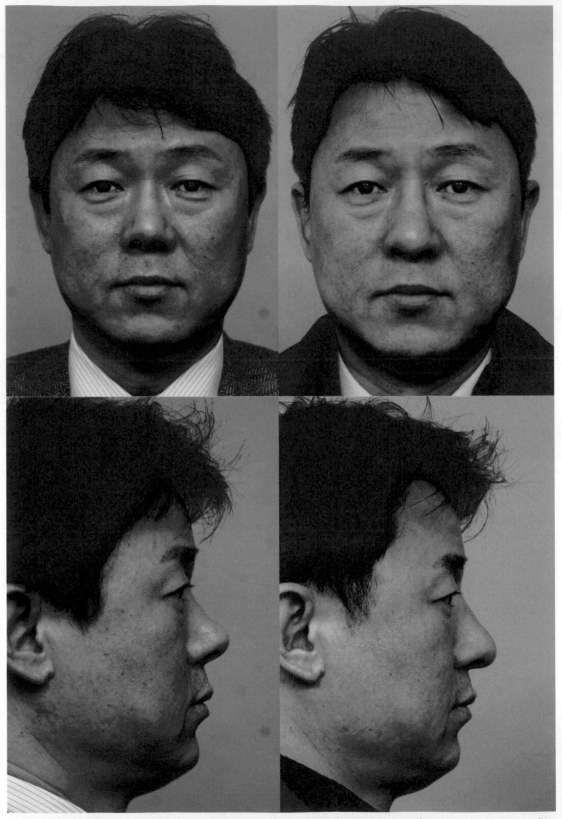

Fig. 24. A patient with a short-nose deformity treated with extended spreader grafting, multilayer tip grafting using conchal cartilage, right lateral crural strut grafting, and dorsal augmentation using ePTFE. Before surgery (*left*), and 6 months after surgery (*right*).

SUMMARY

Similarities and differences exist between rhinoplasties for white and Asian people. In contrast with rhinoplasty for white people, in Asian rhinoplasty, dorsal augmentation is more commonly performed using alloplastic implants. For improvements of the Asian nasal tip, shield grafting, multilayer cartilaginous tip grafting, modified vertical dome division, and tip onlay grafting are invaluable in the rhinoplastic surgeon's armamentarium.

However, as in rhinoplasty for white people, the most difficult surgeries in Asian rhinoplasty involve the correction of deformed noses. Deviated noses and convex dorsum require meticulous analysis of both the nasal framework and facial anatomy. Management of the septum is of particular importance. Short noses also require particular attention in that the appearance of the short nose may be real or perceived, brought about by a disharmony of nasal features. The condition of the skin–soft tissue envelope, especially in revision cases, poses a challenge, particularly in skin closure. Meticulous preoperative assessment, detailed surgical planning with the patient, and preparedness through anticipation of possible complications ensure a satisfactory result for both the patient and the surgeon.

REFERENCES

1. McKinney P, Sweis I. A clinical definition of an ideal nasal radix. Plast Reconstr Surg 2002;109:1416–8.
2. Wang JH, Jang YJ, Park SK, et al. Measurement of aesthetic proportions in the profile view of Koreans. Ann Plast Surg 2009;62:109–13.
3. Kim JS, Khan NA, Song HM, et al. Intraoperative measurements of harvestable septal cartilage in rhinoplasty. Ann Plast Surg 2010;65:519–23.
4. Cho GS, Kim SH, Yeo NK, et al. Nasal skin thickness measured using computed tomography and its effect on tip surgery outcomes. Otolaryngol Head Neck Surg 2011;144:522–7.
5. Jang YJ, Moon BJ. State of the art in augmentation rhinoplasty: implant or graft? Curr Opin Otolaryngol Head Neck Surg 2012;20:280–8.
6. Godin MS, Waldman SR, Johnson CM. Nasal augmentation using Gore-Tex: a 10-year experience. Arch Facial Plast Surg 1999;1:118–21.
7. Jung YJ, Kim HY, Dhong HJ. Ultrasonic monitoring of implant thickness after augmentation rhinoplasty with expanded polytetrafluoroethylene. Am J Rhinol Allergy 2009;23:105–10.
8. Wang JH, Lee BJ, Jang YJ. Use of silicone sheets for dorsal augmentation in rhinoplasty for Asian noses. Acta Otolaryngol Suppl 2007;558:115–20.
9. Daniel RK. Diced cartilage grafts in rhinoplasty surgery: current techniques and applications. Plast Reconstr Surg 2008;122:1883–91.
10. Moon BJ, Lee HJ, Jang YJ. Outcomes following rhinoplasty using autologous costal cartilage. Arch Facial Plast Surg 2012;14:175–80.
11. Wang H, Fan F, You J, et al. Combined silicone implant and cartilage grafts for dorsal augmentation rhinoplasty. J Craniofac Surg 2013;24:494–6.
12. Jang YJ, Min JY, Lau BC. A multilayer cartilaginous tip-grafting technique for improved nasal tip refinement in Asian rhinoplasty. Otolaryngol Head Neck Surg 2011;145:217–22.
13. Yu MS, Jang YJ. Modified vertical dome division technique for rhinoplasty in Asian patients. Laryngoscope 2010;120:668–72.
14. Jang YJ, Kim JH. Use of Tutoplast-processed fascia as an onlay graft material for tip surgery in rhinoplasty. Otolaryngol Head Neck Surg 2011;144(4):528–32.
15. Jang YJ, Yeo NK, Wang JH. Cutting and suture technique of the caudal septal cartilage for the management of caudal septal deviation. Arch Otolaryngol Head Neck Surg 2009;135:1256–60.
16. Kim JH, Kim DY, Jang YJ. Outcomes after endonasal septoplasty using caudal septal batten grafting. Am J Rhinol Allergy 2011;25:166–70.
17. Jang YJ, Kim JM, Yeo NK. Use of nasal septal bone to straighten deviated septal cartilage in correction of deviated nose. Ann Otol Rhinol Laryngol 2009;118:488–94.
18. Jang YJ, Kwon M. Modified extracorporeal septoplasty technique in rhinoplasty for severely deviated noses. Ann Otol Rhinol Laryngol 2010;119:331–5.
19. Cho GS, Jang YJ. Deviated nose correction: different outcomes according to the deviation type. Laryngoscope 2013;123:1136–42.
20. Jang YJ, Kim JH. Classification of convex nasal dorsum deformities in Asian patients and treatment outcomes. J Plast Reconstr Aesthet Surg 2011;64:301–6.
21. Kim SK, Kim HS. Secondary Asian rhinoplasty: lengthening the short nose. Aesthet Surg J 2013;33:353–62.
22. Hyun SM, Jang YJ. Treatment outcomes of saddle nose correction. JAMA Facial Plast Surg 2013;15:280–6.

African American Rhinoplasty

Jennings R. Boyette, MD[a], Fred J. Stucker, MD[b],*

KEYWORDS

- African rhinoplasty • African American rhinoplasty • Black American • Nonwhite • Ethnic rhinoplasty

KEY POINTS

- There is significant variation in nasal anatomy among patients of African descent.
- The goal of surgery is to address only what the patient requests as change to their nose and not to duplicate a preconceived nasal ideal.
- Balance dorsal augmentation with tip projection.
- Avoid excessive alar base narrowing because it can create deformity and disharmony.
- Creating aesthetic refinement while maintaining ethnic features is key to successful surgery.

INTRODUCTION

As the ethnic demographics of the nation continue to evolve so too does the demand for facial plastic surgery among patients of diverse ethnic backgrounds. Today's surgeon must approach each patient as a unique individual with a distinct set of goals for that patient. Patients of African descent who seek out rhinoplasty surgery have similar motives as those of other groups seeking rhinoplasty surgery: to improve nasal aesthetic harmony and nasal function, and not for racial transformation.

In 1976, the senior author published an article concerning the nonwhite rhinoplasty. At that time, there was little in the literature concerning the subject and it was a rare surgeon with significant expertise in this area.[1] Before that time there had been many generalizations and misconceptions reported on the nasal anatomy of those of African descent,[2] and this article advocated for the recognition that most patients do not exhibit all of those anatomic features (**Fig. 1**) and that the goal of each rhinoplasty should be to create harmony in an individual and not to duplicate a preconceived nasal ideal. Since that time, many others have expanded on this conversation and the practice of patient-specific surgery has gained almost universal acceptance.

Now, almost 40 years later, the number of patients of African descent has increased as has the number of facial plastic surgeons who routinely manage these patients. Recent surveys on plastic surgery trends have reported that African Americans constitute 7% to 8% of all plastic surgery patients.[3,4] According to the 2012 American Academy of Facial Plastic Surgery 2012 survey, 27% of surgeons report an increase in African American patients seeking facial plastic surgery and 80% of these patients are seeking rhinoplasty.[5]

PREOPERATIVE CONSULTATION

Unfortunately, insensitivity to a patient's ethnic features, and the well-known disastrous rhinoplasty results of certain celebrities, have created some suspicion and caution among many African American patients. Therefore, it is important to recognize and address any trepidation and

Disclosures: Neither author has any disclosures.
[a] Department of Otolaryngology/Head and Neck Surgery, University of Arkansas for Medical Sciences, 4301 West Markham Street, Slot 543, Little Rock, AR 72205, USA; [b] Department of Otolaryngology/Head and Neck Surgery, Louisiana State University Health Sciences Center—Shreveport, 1501 Kings Highway, Shreveport, LA 71130, USA
* Corresponding author.
E-mail address: fstuck@lsuhsc.edu

Facial Plast Surg Clin N Am 22 (2014) 379–393
http://dx.doi.org/10.1016/j.fsc.2014.04.004

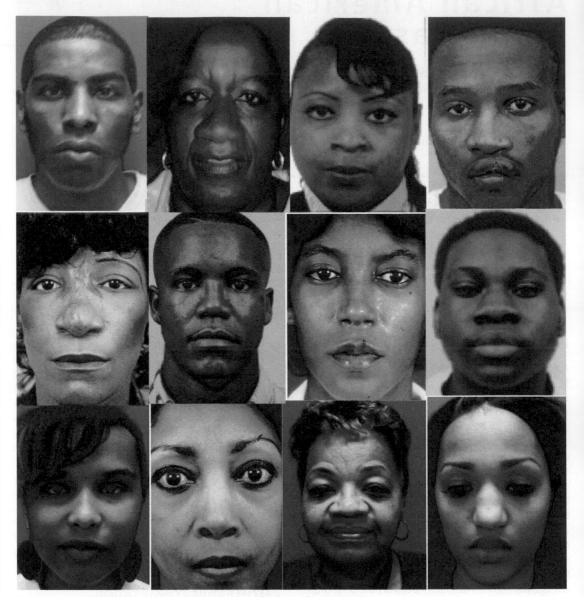

Fig. 1. Composite demonstrating the variations of ethnic characteristics.

misconception in the preoperative visit. Even patients presenting with a nasal bone fracture or a deviated nasal septum often voice concerns about changes to the appearance of their nose. This is the opportunity to establish the necessary rapport with the patient and to let them know that you share their concerns and are sensitive their specific requests for nasal modifications.

The patient should be asked to identify those specific areas that they would like changed. This may be difficult for the patient to express precisely and often it is helpful to use a mirror and have them point out the regions of their nose that they wish to be addressed. Some modifications can even be manually simulated and computer imaging may

be of further assistance. Often the patient states that they just want their nose to "look better." Approach these patients with caution, because their vision of a "better" nose may be incongruous to yours.

At this time, it is appropriate to then point out some of the common anatomic findings in a nose of African descent. You can then balance your nasal analysis with the patient's requests. Be sure to share your findings with the patient. As white surgeons, the authors also find that it is helpful to compare our own noses with the patient's and to point out the differences between the two. Let the patient know that you recognize that everyone's nose need not appear the same, and this often can help allay their concerns and open a dialogue on creating facial harmony.

Although many of our African American patients have similar goals of nasal modification as patients of any other descent (eg, correction of crooked nasal deformity, internal valve collapse, tip ptosis), there are certain requests that are common to this patient population. In their survey of 196 patients, Baker and Krause[6] found that most patients did not want their modifications to resemble white noses and that the most common complaints were that their noses were "too large, too broad, or too wide." Momoh and colleagues[7] report that patients of African descent commonly wish to address specific features: "alar flare, tip definition, dorsal irregularities, and decreased tip projection." Rohrich and Muzaffar[8] describe the goals of African American rhinoplasty to be "maintaining nasal-facial harmony and balance; a narrower, straight dorsum; enhanced tip projection and definition; slight alar flaring; and narrower interalar distance."

Not all patients desire all of these stated goals, nor are they realistically obtainable. For example, many patients only want more tip definition and not a change in their interalar distance. It is important to address only the patient's goals and not the generalized goals of the surgeon. However, even if the patient wants some of these changes addressed, they often do not want these changes taken to the extreme of conforming to a European nasal ideal.

Another concern in the preoperative consultation is the patient who presents desiring radical changes to remove their features that suggest an African heritage. We recommend avoiding surgery in these patients. In the future we may see more patients requesting rhinoplasty to accentuate, and not to hide, their African heritage.

Failure of a patient to clearly identify the changes they wish or a surgeon's failure to realistically appreciate what the patient wants, or whether he or she can realistically achieve those goals, should be absolute indicators not to proceed with surgery. This mature approach often results in these issues being resolved.

GENERAL ANATOMIC CONCERNS

It must be reiterated that patients of African descent do not all share the same nasal anatomy, because there is significant variability among this patient population depending on their own individual heritages. However, there are some general anatomic features that are consistently seen.

The skin is typically thick with an abundance of subcutaneous fibrofatty tissue. This layer often measures between 2 and 4 mm in thickness.[8] This thick soft tissue envelope is especially noticeable in the nasal tip in which the thick skin contributes to the creation of a broad and bulbous appearance. This thickened skin makes it more difficult to see and feel the shape of the lower lateral cartilages (LLCs) through the skin during the preoperative assessment. It is surgically more difficult to create noticeable changes and refinement in the nasal tip.

The size and strength of the LLCs also contribute the wider appearance of the tip. The LLCs in patients of African descent have often been described as being somewhat shorter in total length and more flaccid. However, in a cadaver study conducted by Ofodile and James,[9] the average width and height of the LLCs were reported to be similar in size to that of white noses. However, their study only focused on measurements of the lateral crus.[9] It is likely that a widened alar base gives the appearance of shortened lateral crura in relation to the overall width of the nose. The relationship of the medial crura (which is also thought to be shorter in general) to the lateral crura is more likely responsible for the broad nasal tips commonly seen in patients of African descent. The intradomal angle is often described as large and obtuse, which can lack the sharp, acute definition of the intermediate crus seen in the white nose.[8,10,11] The nasal spine is also less prominent, which translates to even less tip projection.[8,10] The angle of inclination of the LLCs in relation to the plane of the maxilla may also be more acute and cause an underrotation of the tip.[7,10] In patients of African descent, Ofodile and Bokhari[12] reported the average nasolabial angle to be 91 degrees in women and 84 degrees in men (Fig. 2). Contrast these figures to the ideal nasolabial angles ranging from 90 to 105 degrees recommended by most surgeons.

The underlying bony structure also differs. The pyriform aperature is described as wider and more oval in shape.[13] This spreads the base of the nose more lateral, increasing the interalar distance and decreasing nasal projection. Based on anthropometric measurements, Porter[14] found the ratio of intercanthal distance to nasal width to be 1:1.3 in African American men compared with the classically described 1:1 relationship based on the white nose. Excessive alar flare, such that the edge of the ala extends greater than 2 mm lateral to the alar base attachment, is also commonly seen.[8] The shape of the nostrils varies but can often approximate a horizontal orientation. This horizontal orientation moves the classical 2:1 columella to lobule ratio to closer to a 1:1 ratio (Fig. 3).[13]

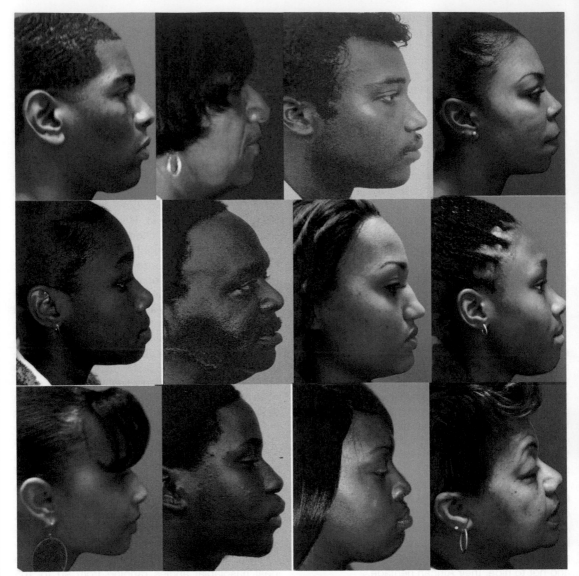

Fig. 2. Multiple lateral views show variations in dorsal height and nasolabial angle. The acute nasolabial angle is the most consistent anatomic finding.

Short nasal bones are commonly encountered.[13] In combination with the widened pyriform aperture and decreased height of the ascending maxilla, these shortened nasal bones create a low and broad nasal dorsum. Therefore, the nasofrontal angle is often more obtuse, 127 to 133 degrees, in comparison with 120 degrees in the white nose.[14,15] These shortened nasal bones and low dorsum may contribute to the authors' observation that nasal bone fractures in patients of African descent often do not result in the visible asymmetries commonly requiring correction in the white nose. There is no doubt that nasal fractures and the subsequent deformities are less common when compared with a comparable white population. Unfortunately, this results in more subtle deformities and often delayed and/or underrecognized abnormalities.

This broad, lowered dorsum also translates down into the upper lateral cartilages, which can result in a broad middle third. These differences may impact nasal function in some patients. As the height of the internal valve is lowered, the shape of the surface area for nasal airflow is placed more inferiorly and centered more on the head of the inferior turbinate. Thus, the inferior turbinates have a more significant role in nasal obstructive symptoms in patients with this nasal anatomy.[16]

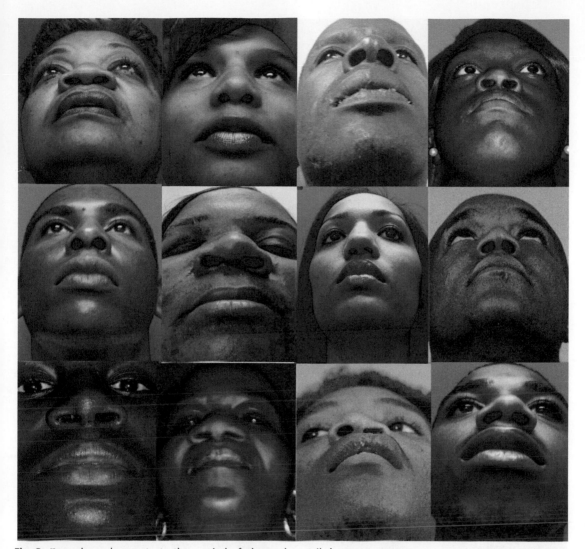

Fig. 3. Base views demonstrate the myriad of alar and nostril shapes.

SURGICAL TECHNIQUES

Whether to use an endonasal technique or perform an external approach is essentially dictated by the changes sought, the preference of the surgeon, and the patient's concerns. Another important consideration is the potential for surgical change in the individual patient. Some preoperative maneuvers answer these questions (**Fig. 4**). The authors' personal philosophy for all nasal surgery is to use the least complex technique that permits accomplishing the desired changes. Many surgeons prefer to use an external approach in patients of African descent.[7,8,17,18] We also find that the increased exposure afforded by the external approach allows for creation of the more dramatic changes that are often necessary in the nose of patients of African descent. However, routine tip

surgery can still be accomplished by way of an endonasal approach. The placement of a columellar strut, which is one of the most common maneuvers used in these patients, can easily be placed by way of an endonasal technique (**Fig. 5**). As a general rule, if a tip graft is contemplated, then an external approach with a transcolumellar incision is used.

In the past some surgeons have raised concern over the transcolumellar incision in keloid-prone patients; however, in more than 500 rhinoplasties in African American patients, the senior author has not observed keloid formation in this area. Other authors have noted this rarity of keloid occurrence.[8,18,19] It is worth noting that the decortication involved in an external rhinoplasty may increase the postoperative rounding of the tip secondary to spherical scarring. This scarring may actually help to narrow the tip and create a

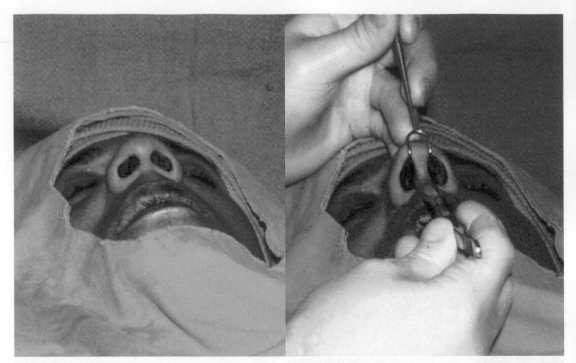

Fig. 4. These preoperative maneuvers indicate whether certain surgical changes will occur without the telltale surgical look or an incongruous appearance.

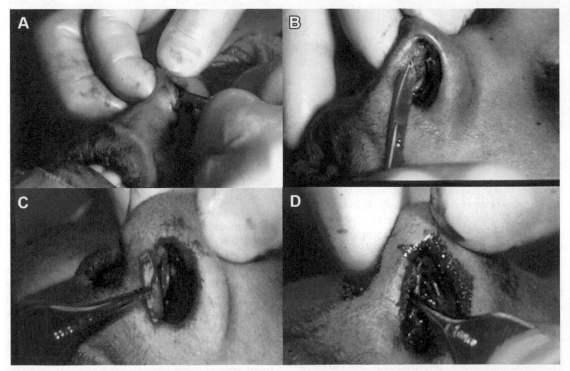

Fig. 5. Placement of a columellar strut through an endonasal approach. (*A*) Vertical 5- to 8-mm incision through skin behind medial crura. (*B*) Pocket developed between medial crurae and separate intradomal fibers. (*C*) Sizing the septal cartilage strut. (*D*) Placement of strut, closure should include fixation of graft and both medial crurae (mattress suture).

subtle increase in projection without the need for additional tip grafts. Additionally, in patients with a very short columella, lengthening can be achieved by using the transcolumellar incision to create a V to Y advancement flap at the columellar base (**Fig. 6**).

The key to successful rhinoplasty in these patients is to balance each modification to achieve the patient's goals without attempting large-scale nasal changes. Thus, rhinoplasty in the nose of African descent may often be a much more subtle surgery than that performed in the white nose. The individual techniques often used to achieve this balance are increasing tip projection and definition, augmentation of the dorsum, and reduction of alar base width and flare. Many surgeons have reported on these three modifications as the ones most commonly used in noses of African descent.[7,8,10,17,19,20]

NASAL DORSUM

Although many patients of African descent present with an underprojected nasal dorsum, this is

certainly not the rule. In fact, in the senior author's early series 23% of patients presented with a dorsal hump.[1] In either case, it is necessary to balance the projection of dorsum with the projection of the tip. Even the most markedly deficient nasal dorsal height should not be augmented if there is insufficient tip projection to achieve harmony. A nasal dorsum that is augmented beyond what the tip projection can accommodate loses its aesthetic proportions. This harmony transcends any nasal measurements (**Fig. 7**).

The authors agree with Harris[20] that "a high dorsum is not essential for a continuous brow-tip aesthetic line," and that a low nasal bridge can often be aesthetically pleasing in relation to the patients other features. Excessive augmentation of the nasal dorsum in the patient of African descent should be avoided, because it may result in racial incongruity.[20] Therefore, consider augmenting the dorsum to remain slightly underprojected compared with the white nose. A subtle augmentation to create highlights in the skin along the brow-aesthetic line is often enough to eliminate the "washed out" bridge that patients often want corrected, and create the illusion of dorsal narrowing (**Fig. 8**). Because the amount of dorsal augmentation is most often limited by the extent of nasal tip projection that can be reasonably achieved, it is the authors' practice and recommendation to establish tip projection before augmentation of the dorsum.

Successful augmentation has been reported with a variety of graft materials. Rohrich and Muzaffar[8] reported on using septal cartilage onlay grafts to achieve less than 2 mm of augmentation, acellular cadaveric dermis to achieve 2 to 5 mm of

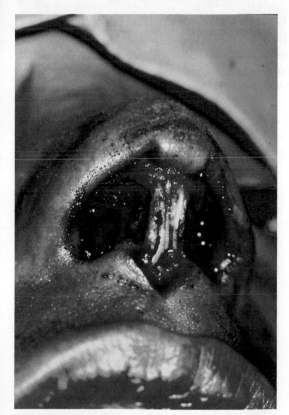

Fig. 6. V-shaped incision at the base of the columella, which can then be closed as a Y to recruit columellar length. A mattress suture through the medial crura flare aids in the closure and recruitment of additional tissue into the columella.

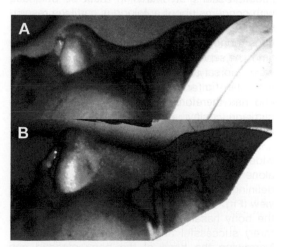

Fig. 7. (A) Performing the tip surgery first allows for a more accurate assessment of the degree of appropriate dorsal augmentation. (B) Six millimeters of increased dorsal height.

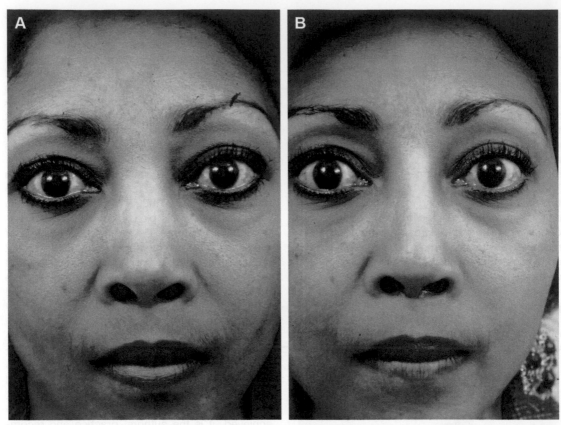

Fig. 8. Dorsal augmentation with a thin strip of expanded polytetrafluoroethylene, which improves the preoperative "washed out" look. Before (*A*) and after dorsal augmentation (*B*).

augmentation, and costal cartilage for more than 5 mm of augmentation. Others have reported good results with expanded polytetrafluoroethylene or porous polyethylene.[17,20] Concerns about infection and graft extrusion must be balanced with concerns about autologous cartilage resorption. Reported figures regarding graft complications range from 1.9% to 20% (**Fig. 9**).[21,22] Over time, the senior author has favored a more conservative dorsal augmentation to maintain harmony with the tip and to maintain ethnic features, and has therefore found the use of autologous cartilage onlay grafts to provide sufficient augmentation.

The width of the nasal dorsum can often appear widened in these patients. Dorsal augmentation alone typically improves this appearance by better defining the dorsal aesthetic highlights on frontal view (**Fig. 10**).[23] The use of osteotomies to narrow the bony nasal dorsum as a single maneuver is rarely successful and is generally discouraged. Narrowing the base of the bony pyramid can create an incongruity between the dorsum and the remainder of the widened central facial structures. However, if there is deformity or asymmetry

of the nasal bones, then osteotomies are certainly recommended.

TIP SURGERY

A moderate increase in tip projection and a refinement of the tip is the most common goal in patients of African descent. An acute nasolabial angle is usually encountered and some patients request rotation of the tip. It should be noted that goals of tip contouring, surface aesthetics, and well-defined tip-defining points that are commonly discussed in rhinoplasty are often difficult to achieve in the patient of African descent. It should be reiterated that these patients typically have thick skin and round, full nasal lobules that mask the structure of the LLCs through the skin. Skeletonizing and narrowing the tip to create the surface aesthetics of a thin-skinned white nose may result in a disharmony and racial transformation.

Several strategies can be used to increase projection, definition, and rotation, such as domal suture techniques, crural steal, columellar strut/septal extension grafting, and tip grafting. A combination of some or all of the above is commonly

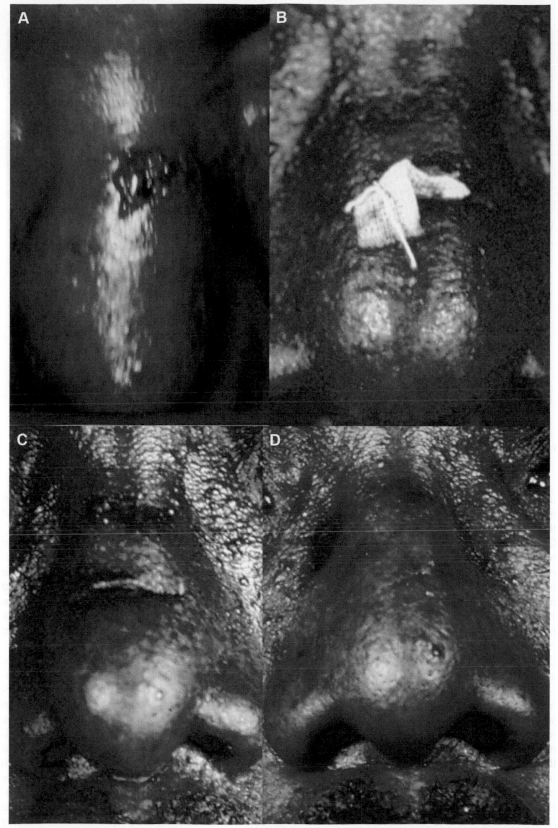

Fig. 9. (*A*) Patient with extruding proplast implant. (*B*) One week postoperative before removal of iodoform wick. (*C*) Two months after removal of implant through extruded site. (*D*) One year after revision with Z-plasty.

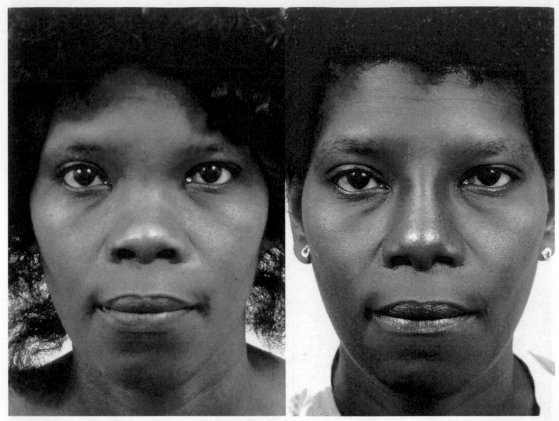

Fig. 10. Dorsal augmentation can give an apparent appearance of decreasing the alar width.

used. In agreement with Harris,[20] the authors also advocate for a "ground up" approach—building the tip projection from the nasal spine upward. Others have also noted that the premaxilla and nasal spine are often less developed in the patient of African descent.[10] Therefore, a columellar strut is routinely fashioned from the septal cartilage and used to add tip support and project the tip. The cartilaginous septum may be short and relatively thin; however, there is generally sufficient cartilage for columellar strut and a tip graft. Correction of an actual septal deformity is required in less than 10% of patients.[11]

In addition to the columellar strut, suture techniques can then be used to further increase projection and narrow the tip. In some patients the medial crura may be elongated, causing columellar flare into the nasal vestibule. In these patients a medial crural steal technique can be used to attach the crura to the columellar strut, narrowing the columella and increasing projection. Patients of African descent often have a widely divergent angle at the intermediate crus. Therefore, lateral crural steal is often a good option for increasing projection.[10] However, the lateral crura

may be short and too much lateral crural steal can create a flaccid external valve in these patients (if additional support is not added).[10,24]

Interdomal sutures can also be used to increase projection and are commonly used in concert with a columellar strut. The divergence between the medial and lateral crura can then be narrowed with intradomal sutures to increase definition. The senior author has also described a technique of intradomal suturing endonasally in the patient of African descent (**Fig. 11**).[1]

If suture techniques do not accomplish the desired changes in the tip, additional graft augmentation can be performed. Because of the thick overlying skin envelope, these onlay grafts are often needed if significant projection and definition is necessary. The type of graft depends on the individual needs of the patient. Rohrich advocates that Gunter (combined infratip lobular and onlay tip) grafts are best suited for these patients, because the tip and the infratip regions benefit from augmentation.[8] These grafts can also be stacked in multiple layers to further increase projection.[8,10,20] We only use stacked grafts that have a significant amount of adherent perichondrium.

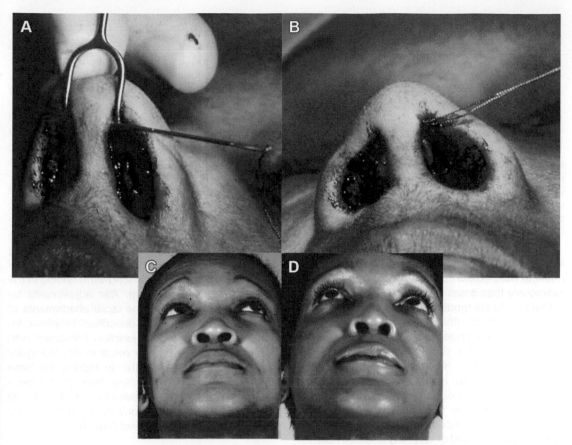

Fig. 11. Superior bunching suture technique of placing a domal binding suture. (*A*) Placement is aided with a ball retractor. (*B*) Effect of suture placement. (*C*) Preoperative and (*D*) 1-year postoperative views.

Underrotation of the tip is also commonly encountered in the patient of African descent. Increases in rotation can be performed with the columellar strut and interdomal sutures; however, further techniques, such as lateral crural overlay, may also be needed. Many of these patients have a hypoplastic premaxilla, which can result in columellar retraction and accentuate the appearance of underrotation. Premaxillary and columellar plumping grafts can create a less acute nasolabial angle.[11,24] Severing or preferably stripping the attachments of the depressor septi allows superior rotation and also can help to prevent this muscle from exerting a downward pull on the tip in the early postoperative period. Over the years the long-term corrections of the acute nasolabial angle is one of the most refractory to correction and is prone to relapse.

The increased thickness of the soft tissue over the tip has led many surgeons to practice soft tissue thinning and defatting as a way to further refine the tip. Rohrich and Muzaffar[8] suggest only removing the excess fibrofatty tissue directly over the dome. Harris[20] leaves the fibrofatty tissue

pedicled inferiorly and transposes it into the infratip region for increased bulk and contour at that region. Any type of thinning should be done with caution and with care to avoid the subdermal plexus. Although thinning may create more definition to the tip, this definition may also remove the characteristic rounding of the tip that is associated with African heritage. Defatting and aggressive attempts to thin the skin are discouraged and fraught with pigmented changes.

ALAR BASE

Many patients request a narrower alar base. However, nasal base modifications are likely overused and are frequently responsible for the creation of a surgical-appearing nose and nasal disharmony in the patient of African descent. We must recognize that the ideal alar position and width is different from the white ideal. Furthermore, a recent study by Bennett and colleagues[25] reported that the long-term effect of alar base reduction was essentially a relapse to the preoperative width. Therefore, because alar base reduction may be of little

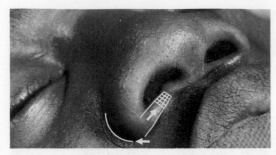

Fig. 12. Recommended placement of incision. Never place incision on the anterior face of the cheek (*asterisk*). Place alar base incision internally, in the sill area or on the lateral ala approximately 1 mm superior to the melolabial crease before ala surgery (*arrows*).

long-term value and may result in noticeable scarring and nostril deformities, it should be used more judiciously than it has in the past.

Most alar base modifications cannot be properly assessed until all other steps have been carried out. Gaining tip projection often markedly influences the proportion of nasal width to height. Rohrich and Muzaffar[8] recommend addressing the alar base if alar flare extends greater than 2 mm. Harris reports that patents with a horizontally oriented nostril benefit from alar wedge resection and nasal base reduction much more than those patients with inverted or vertically oriented nostrils.

The most common maneuver the authors perform is the medialization of the alar base without the benefit of an incision along the alar base. The sill is mobilized by placing a small incision along the inferior crease. A second incision is placed, running roughly parallel, approximately 5 mm intransasally. The entire ala is mobilized, but the skin of the lateral meloalar crease is intact. Occasionally the recruited skin from the floor can

be used for columellar deficiency. More commonly the medialized excess skin is resected at the medial aspect of the sill (**Fig. 12**). The ala is advanced, and a deep permanent suture purchases the subcutaneous tissue, the sill dermis, and its mate on the opposite ala, thus cinching the ala together (**Fig. 13**).

Alar base reduction must also be performed judiciously to avoid narrowing the nasal base too much in proportion to the wide nasal dorsum and broad nasal tip. A gradual decrease in alar flare can satisfy the patient without resulting in racial incongruity. It is important to counsel the patient preoperatively as to reasonable expectations for nasal base reduction. Aggressive alar base surgery can often result in a triangular tip in base view where the ala no longer have a slight curving flare just superior to the alar-facial junction. Unfortunately, this is a common long-term finding in the patient of African descent. Alar adjustments by separating the ala from the facial attachments at the groove are commonly described. However, incisions at the alar-facial junction combined with alar resections can easily result in this triangular deformity. It is much better to reduce the base through resections in the nasal floor, thus preserving the curvature of the nostril margin. It is difficult to achieve absolute harmony when very large alar base resections are required (**Fig. 14**).

SUMMARY

There are some major changes in the global view of the topic of African American rhinoplasty over the past 40 years. The most obvious changes are the number of patients seeking surgery and the number of surgeons experienced and comfortable in managing these cases. Another notable change to the senior author is the acceptability of the

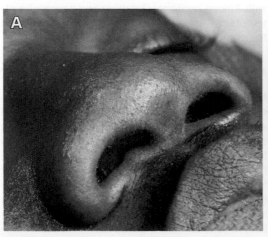
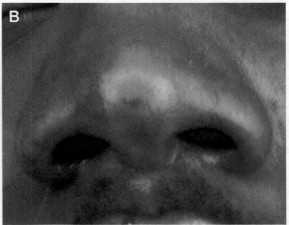

Fig. 13. Sill resection and medialization before (*A*) and after (*B*) deep dermal sutures have been placed.

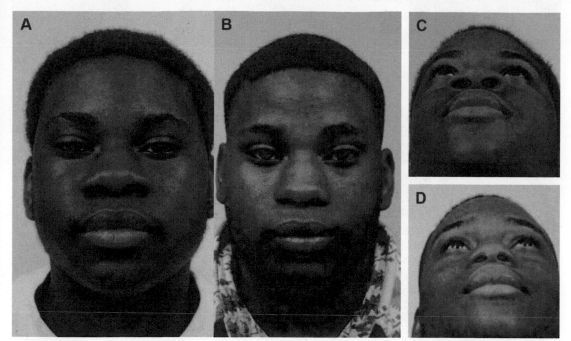

Fig. 14. (*A*) Preoperative full face view. (*B*) Four years postoperative of 1 cm × 2 cm wedge resection of alar base. (*C*) Preoperative base view. (*D*) Postoperative view indicates lack of natural curve of the alar base.

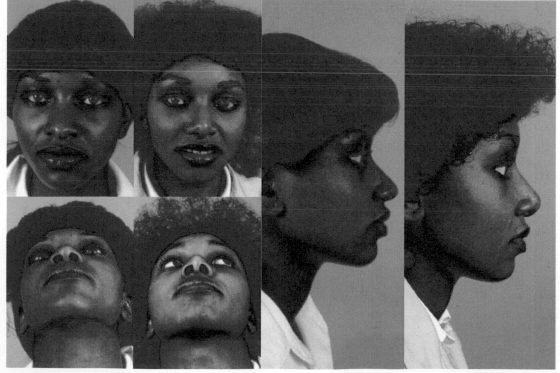

Fig. 15. Composite of patient having undergone endonasal dome-binding with superior bunching sutures (the "cloud" approach).

392

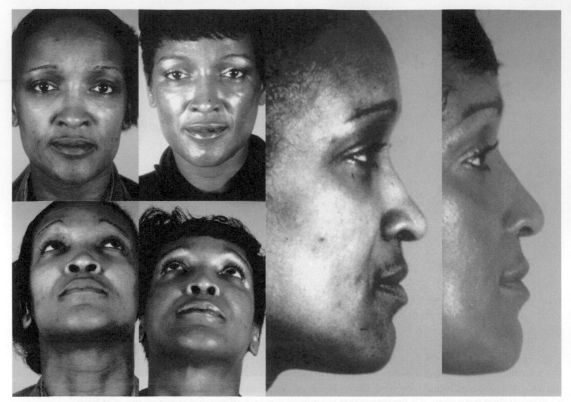

Fig. 16. Preoperative and postoperative photographs. Surgery used the base of columella external approach (2 years postoperative).

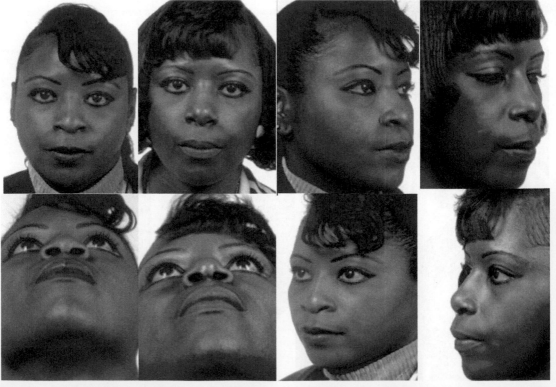

Fig. 17. Composite of preoperative and postoperative photographs using the typical midcolumellar incision (2 years postoperative).

African American male to pursue surgery on their nose.

A steady change noted is the sophistication of all patients who are pursuing nasal surgery. Patients are more able to articulate exactly what changes they desire. Forty years from now we suspect that the topic of nonwhite rhinoplasty will be obsolete, and the issues of the patient's desires and the surgical anatomic manipulation will prevail.

There are instances when adjunctive procedures, such as mentoplasty and reduction cheiloplasty, enhance the overall improvement. It is extremely important to discuss these ancillary procedures with the patient because many are unaware of these procedures, or reluctant to undergo these changes. We continue to recommend the simplest procedure that addresses the correction desired. Subtle changes, an "unoperated" look, and harmony are the hallmarks of surgery in the African American nose (**Figs. 15–17**).

REFERENCES

1. Stucker FJ. Non-caucasian rhinoplasty. Trans Sect Otolaryngol Am Acad Ophthalmol Otolaryngol 1976;82(4):417–22.
2. Schultz AH. Relation of the external nose to the bony nose and nasal cartilages in whites and negroes. Am J Phys Anthropol 1913;1:329.
3. American Society of Plastic Surgeons. National Clearinghouse of Plastic Surgery Statistics. Available at: http://www.plasticsurgery.org/Documents/news-resources/statistics/2012-Plastic-Surgery-Statistics/full-plastic-surgery-statistics-report.pdf. Accessed December 13, 2013.
4. Cosmetic Surgery National Data Bank Statistics. 2012. Available at: http://www.surgery.org/sites/default/files/ASAPS-2012-Stats.pdf. Accessed December 13, 2013.
5. American Academy of Facial Plastic Surgery 2012 membership survey. Available at: http://www.aafprs.org/wp-content/themes/aafprs/pdf/AAFPRS-2012-REPORT.pdf. Accessed December 13, 2013.
6. Baker HL, Krause CJ. Update on the negroid nose: an anatomic and anthropometric analysis. In: Ward PH, Berman WE, editors. Plastic and reconstructive surgery of the head and neck: Proceedings of the Fourth International Symposium. 1st edition. St Louis (MO): Mosby; 1984. p. 85–93.
7. Momoh AO, Hatef DA, Griffin A, et al. Rhinoplasty: the African American patient. Semin Plast Surg 2009;23(3):223–31.
8. Rohrich RJ, Muzaffar AR. Rhinoplasty in the African-American patient. Plast Reconstr Surg 2003;111(3):1322–39.
9. Ofodile FA, James EA. Anatomy of alar cartilages in blacks. Plast Reconstr Surg 1997;100(3):699–703.
10. Chike-Obi CJ, Boahene K, Bullocks JM, et al. Tip nuances for the nose of African descent. Facial Plast Surg 2012;28(2):194–201.
11. Stucker FJ, Lian T, Sanders K. African American rhinoplasty. Facial Plast Surg Clin North Am 2005;13(1):65–72.
12. Ofodile FA, Bokhari F. The African-American nose: part II. Ann Plast Surg 1995;34(2):123–9.
13. Ofodile FA. Nasal bones and pyriform apertures in blacks. Ann Plast Surg 1994;32(1):21–6.
14. Porter JP. The average African American male face: an anthropometric analysis. Arch Facial Plast Surg 2004;6(2):78–81.
15. Porter JP, Olson KL. Analysis of the African American female nose. Plast Reconstr Surg 2003;111(2):620–6.
16. Zhu JH, Lee HP, Kim KM, et al. Evaluation and comparison of nasal airway flow patterns among three subjects from Caucasian, Chinese, and Indian ethnic groups using computational fluid dynamics simulation. Respir Physiolo Neurobiol 2011;175:62–9.
17. Romo T, Presti P. Aesthetic reconstruction of the platyrrhine nose. In: Stucker FJ, de Souza C, Kenyon GS, et al, editors. Rhinology and facial plastic surgery. 1st edition. New York: Springer; 2009. p. 761–8.
18. Patrocinio LG, Patrocinio JA. Open rhinoplasty for African-American noses. Br J Oral Maxillofac Surg 2007;45(7):561–6.
19. Slupchynskyj O, Gieniusz M. Rhinoplasty for African American patients: a retrospective review of 75 cases. Arch Facial Plast Surg 2008;10(4):232–6.
20. Harris MO. Rhinoplasty in the patient of African descent. Facial Plast Surg Clin North Am 2010;18(1):189–99.
21. Conrad K, Torgerson CS, Gillman GS. Applications of Gore-tex implants in rhinoplasty reexamined after 17 years. Arch Facial Plast Surg 2008;10(4):224–31.
22. Mendelsohn M, Dunlop G. Gore-tex augmentation grafting in rhinoplasty—is it safe? J Otolaryngol 1998;27(6):337–41.
23. Hubbard TJ. Bridge narrowing in ethnic noses. Ann Plast Surg 1998;40(3):214–8.
24. Kontis TC, Papel ID. Rhinoplasty on the African-American nose. Aesthetic Plast Surg 2002;26(Suppl 1):S12.
25. Bennett GH, Lessow A, Song P, et al. The long-term effects of alar base reduction. Arch Facial Plast Surg 2005;7(2):94–7.

Rhinoplasty in the Mestizo Nose

Roxana Cobo, MD

KEYWORDS

- Mestizo rhinoplasty • Bulbous nasal tip • Thick skin • Mestizo nose • Hispanic patient
- Mesorrhine nose

KEY POINTS

- Rhinoplasty in Mestizo patients is evolving from reductive aggressive techniques to those whereby a structural stepwise approach is used.
- Mestizo patients want smaller noses that look more defined, while retaining ethnic features.
- The structural technique involves using sutures and grafts to give additional support and create definition with minimal tissue resection.
- Structural grafting involves using cartilage grafts as devices that give additional support to underlying support structures of the nose.
- Sutures are an excellent alternative to increase rotation and create definition without decreasing the support of the nasal tip.

 A video of a septal extension graft accompanies this article at http://www.facialplastic.theclinics.com/

INTRODUCTION

More than half of the growth of the population of the United States from 2000 to 2010 was due to an increase in the Hispanic population.[1] Even though today Hispanics are not the fastest growing ethnic group within the United States, they still are the biggest ethnic minority, making it a very important group of patients seeking facial plastic surgery procedures.

Rhinoplasty is the leading facial plastic procedure that is performed worldwide and Latin America is not an exception.[2] Today there is an increasing awareness that rhinoplasty is not a "one-size-fits-all" procedure and more often more patients are looking for specialists who have experience in dealing with ethnic patients and their particular problems.

The trends in rhinoplasty surgery have also shifted from the traditional reductive aggressive procedures to those wherein ethnic features are preserved. Mestizo patients are not the exception. A structural stepwise approach is presented whereby satisfactory long-term results can be achieved using sutures and graft to reinforce support structures and define nasal features.

THE MESTIZO PATIENT

Mestizo means mixture of races. It is a combination of the local Indian tribes that inhabited the different regions of the continent, the Europeans (mainly Spanish invasions) who initially conquered the area in the fifteenth century, and the Africans that were brought over during the slave trade (**Fig. 1**). Additional European migrations during the first and second World Wars complete the picture.[3]

Mestizo nasal and facial characteristics vary frequently because much depends on which of the different races predominate in the patient's features. In general, the Mestizo nose could be

No disclosures.
Service of Otolaryngology, Centro Médico Imbanaco, Carrera 38A #5A-100 cons 231A, Cali 760044, Colombia
E-mail address: rcobo@imbanaco.com.co

Facial Plast Surg Clin N Am 22 (2014) 395–415
http://dx.doi.org/10.1016/j.fsc.2014.04.011

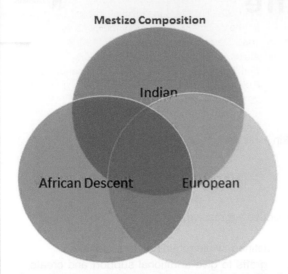

Mestizo Composition

Indian

African Descent   European

Fig. 1. Mestizo racial composition. Mestizos is defined as a mixture of races. In Latin America, it is a combination of Caucasians, African descendants, and local Indian tribes. The proportion will vary depending on the area from where the patient is coming from.

classified as having messorhine characteristics (**Table 1**). The underlying cartilaginous and bony framework is frequently weak with a covering (skin–soft tissue envelope [S-STE]) that tends to be thick, resulting in an external appearance that shows a nose that is bulbous and undefined and

Table 1
Nasal characteristics in Mestizo patients

Nasal Characteristics	Mestizo Patients
Skin type	Normal/thick/sebaceous
S-STE	Thick/tendency toward inflammation
Nasal bones	Normal to short
Bony dorsum	Normal to low radix Wide nasal bridge Small pseudohump
Cartilaginous nasal vault	Normal to weak, wide
Nasal tip/alar cartilages	Flimsy/unsupportive/ wide/undefined Poor tip recoil
Columella	Normal to short
Nasolabial angle	Normal to acute
Nasal spine	Normal to short
Nostril shape	Horizontal shape/ sometimes flaring
Alar base	Normal to wide

can look slightly flattened (**Fig. 2**). Mestizo patients are also known as "Hispanics" and "Latinos" and the 3 terms can sometimes be used interchangeably, although the term Mestizo is the one that most closely defines racial features.[4]

DEFINITION OF PROBLEMS/PLANNING THE SURGERY

A stepwise approach is usually used when planning a rhinoplasty procedure (**Fig. 3**).

1. Patient's desires/definition on what is beautiful to patient

The big question when performing Mestizo rhinoplasty is, what do patients want? In the author's experience, Mestizo patients want smaller noses with more defined-looking features.

2. Cultural/ethnic/racial variations

Latin American Mestizos do not have a specific racial pattern. Individual facial and nasal features will be defined on particular migration patterns of the geographic area from where the patient is coming from. Today, Mestizo patients are considered mixed race patients wherein a blending of characteristics is what can be found as a predominant facial feature.

3. Physical examination/anatomic diagnosis/definition of problems

An accurate physical examination to try to make a correct diagnosis of the different anatomic structures of the nose will let the surgeon establish in an efficient way the different findings of the nose. In this way, a precise definition of the different problems can be established to be able to define what type of solutions can be offered.

4. Photographic documentation

Six standard rhinoplasty views are routinely taken on all patients: front view, base view, left lateral view, left oblique view, right lateral view, right oblique view. These images are used to perform computer imaging with the patient where possible cosmetic results are shown to try and define if they fit with the patient's desires of what he or she wants with their nose. When working with computer imaging, it is very important to show patients realistic images of the changes that can be obtained. Preoperative images are used during surgery and they become an integral part of the patient's medical record. They are constantly used during postoperative visits to show patients how their results are evolving. Postoperative pictures are again taken at 6 months and

1 year after surgery and if possible every year thereafter. This systematic documentation helps evaluate long-term results and aids the surgeon in evaluating surgical techniques used.

5. Discussion of surgical and nonsurgical options

Depending on the patient's physical findings, possible surgical options must be discussed and clarified. It is important for patients to understand the limitations and the existing risks of the surgical procedure that is being offered. The final result ideally should be a patient who is happy with his final result and a surgeon who is happy with the type of surgery he performed and the result obtained.

As mentioned above, patients usually want noses that look smaller and more defined. Anatomically, surgeons are frequently faced with noses that have very poor underlying cartilaginous and bony support structures and a thick S-STE. Surgery should be oriented toward reinforcing support structures of the nose and creating definition of nasal dorsum and tip without resulting in a nose that looks big or bulky.

STRUCTURAL APPROACH IN THE MESTIZO NOSE

When performing rhinoplasty in Mestizo patients, the author has used a structural approach for more than 20 years to tailor the surgery depending on the patient's individual needs. All procedures are done under general anesthesia and generally an open approach is used. The philosophy behind this structural approach is as follows:

- Conservative tissue excision
- Preservation and reinforcement of support structures of the nose
- Structural grafting to reinforce and increase strength of existing anatomic structures
- Precision grafting and filling and exact suture placement to define nasal structures

To help plan the surgery accordingly, the nose is divided into anatomic thirds. Specific techniques are planned for each area and cartilage grafting is planned depending on the needs of each individual patient.

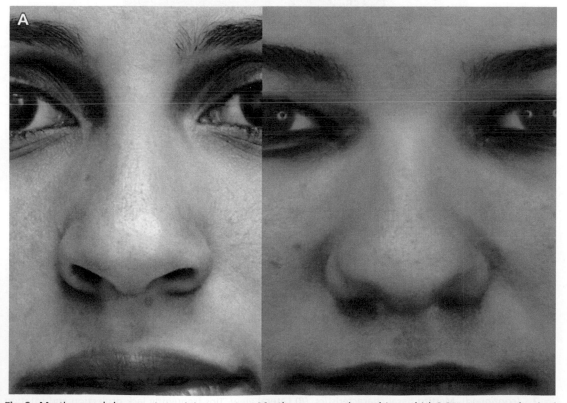

Fig. 2. Mestizo nasal characteristics. (*A*) Front view. Mestizo noses can have thin to thick S-STE. Noses tend to look slightly flattened and small and bones can be relatively short. Tips look wide and have poor definition.

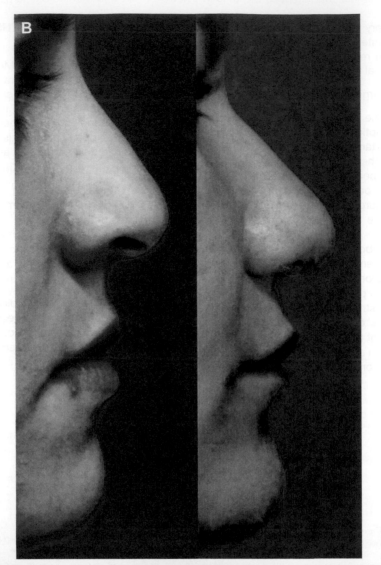

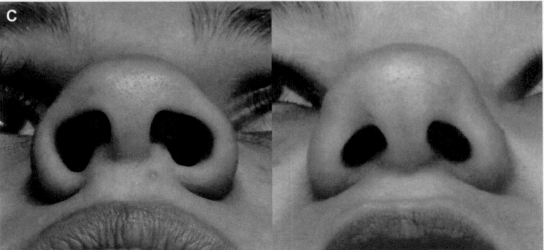

Fig. 2. (*continued*). Mestizo nasal characteristics. (*B*) Lateral view. Tips frequently lack projection and rotation and it is common to find acute nasolabial angles. (*C*) Base view. The nasal base can be wide, slightly flaring, with columellas that have a tendency to be short.

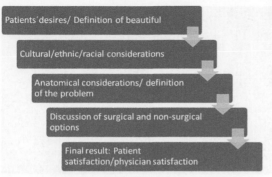

Fig. 3. Stepwise approach in Mestizo rhinoplasty. A structured stepwise approach should always be used wherein patients' desires and ethnic and cultural variations are taken into account when planning the surgery to try and obtain satisfactory final results.

- Upper third of the nose (bony dorsum)
- Middle third of the nose (cartilaginous dorsum)
- Lower third of the nose (nasal tip)

The upper and middle third of the nose (including osteotomies) are usually managed before final tip procedures are performed (**Tables 2** and **3**).

SURGICAL TECHNIQUE

All surgeries are done under general anesthesia. The nose is infiltrated using 1% to 2% Xilocaine + epinephrine 1:100,000.

Harvesting of Cartilage

The first choice for cartilage grafting is the nasal septum. In Mestizo patients, because of the mesorrhine configuration of their nose, the quadrangular cartilage is not very big and is usually not thicker than 2 to 3 mm. This small amount of cartilage is a big limitation because the amount of

Table 3
Gradual approach to the nasal tip

Anatomic Problem	Surgical Solution
Intact strip procedures	
Wide alar cartilage	Cephalic trim of lateral crura
	Lateral crural turn in flap
Suture defining techniques	Lateral crural steal
	Dome-defining sutures
	Lateral crural spanning sutures
	Septocolumellar suture
Incomplete strip procedures	
Overprojected tip/ long plunging nose	Lateral crural overlay technique
	Medial crural overlay technique
Grafts on the nasal tip	
Grafts that increase support and create definition	Shield graft
	Lateral crural strut graft
	Alar rim grafts
	Morcelized cartilage over nasal tip

cartilage available for grafting can sometimes be limited. It becomes imperative to harvest the cartilage as a complete block, leaving at least 1.5 cm caudally and dorsally and leaving a complete inverted L of septum in the nose that will be an important support after surgery. Access to the nasal septum can be gained using a Killian or a caudal septal incision. All deviations are straightened as much as possible, especially those present caudally. The septum is closed using a continuous mattress absorbable suture (**Fig. 4**).[5]

The Open Approach

An inverted V incision is placed at the mid-columellar region immediately above the feet of the medial crura and extending laterally 2 mm behind the crura. Cuts are done perpendicular to the skin, using a no. 15 blade. Laterally, the incision is extended superiorly following the caudal of the intermediate crura and lateral crura.

The flap is elevated using converse scissors, keeping the dissection plane below the musculoaponeurotic system and immediately above the cartilaginous structures of the nasal tip. Once the nasal tip has been dissected, the dissection moves to the midline, elevating the skin over the

Table 2
Surgical solutions to problems in the dorsum and middle third of the nose

Problem	Surgical Solution
Wide dorsum no hump	Medial and lateral osteotomies
Low radix/small pseudohump	Radix graft
Low dorsum	Dorsal augmentation
Weak ULC	Spreader grafts
	Mattress flaring sutures
	Onlay grafts

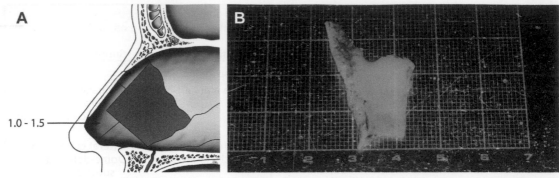

Fig. 4. Harvesting septal cartilage. (*A*) Septal cartilage is always the first choice of grafting material when performing rhinoplasty. An inverted "L" strip of at least 1.0 to 1.5 cm of cartilage should remain to be able to guarantee a stable foundation. (*B*) Image of harvested septal cartilage.

cartilaginous middle third of the nose, directly over the perichondrium, and after the nasal bones are identified, the dissection is done subperiosteally all the way up to the nasofrontal angle (**Fig. 5**).

The Upper Third of the Nose (Bony Dorsum)

In Mestizo patients, nasal bones tend to be short and somewhat flattened. Anatomically common findings are as follows:

a. Wide nasal dorsum without hump

- Surgical technique: medial and lateral osteotomies

  Medial and lateral osteotomies will help narrow a wide dorsum without changing the dorsal height. Medial osteotomies are done first using a 3- to 4-mm curved osteotome. The osteotomy is started in the midline at the junction of the dorsal edge of the septum and the bony dorsum. The osteotome is angled 20 to 30° off the midline to avoid the thick frontal bone. Lateral osteotomies are performed using

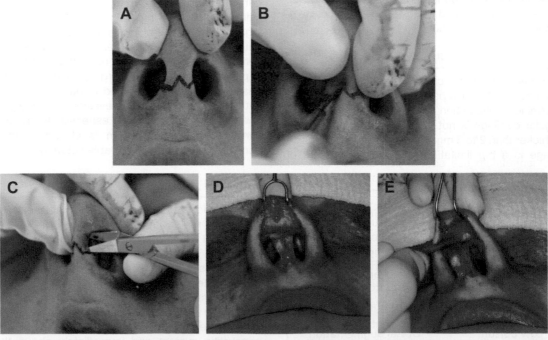

Fig. 5. Open approach. (*A*) Inverted "V" incision marked in the mid-columellar area directly above the feet of the medial crura. (*B*) Incision is done with a no. 15 blade in a perpendicular fashion. (*C, D*) The flap is elevated using converse or Walter's scissors. The dissection plane is kept directly above cartilaginous structures of the nose. (*E*) The dissection is extended subperiosteally all the way up to the nasofrontal angle.

a 2.2-mm guarded osteotome using a high-low-high technique (**Fig. 6**).

b. Shallow radix with small hump or pseudohump
- Surgical technique: radix graft with or without hump reduction

Bony dorsal humps can be lowered using graded rasps, osteotomes, or both. The cartilaginous portion of the hump is lowered using a no. 15 blade and re-secting small slivers of cartilage until the dorsum is smooth. Radix grafts are commonly used to fill in the small con-cavity that is seen in Mestizo patients. A precise pocket is fashioned when elevating the dorsal flap and the space is filled in with crushed cartilage. This pocket helps elevate the dorsal height without the need of bigger grafts or im-plants. Many times a combination of techniques are used: conservative dor-sal rasping with crushed cartilage in the radix to obtain a smooth dorsum with adequate height (**Fig. 7**).[6]

c. Low nasal dorsum
- Surgical technique: dorsal augmentation with cartilage or implants

When dorsal augmentation is needed, this ideally should be performed with cartilage. The author's first choice is always septal cartilage over auricular cartilage. In special cases, rib cartilage can be used when no other cartilage is available. When patients refuse rib cartilage and the available cartilage from septum or concha is not enough, implants can be an option. The author has used expanded polytetrafluoro-ethylene (Gore-Tex) sheeting for more than 20 years with a very low compli-cation rate and excellent results. The implant material should be soaked in antibiotic solution, placed in a precise pocket over the dorsum, and fixed with sutures to the cartilaginous middle third of the nose to avoid shifting (**Fig. 8**).[7,8]

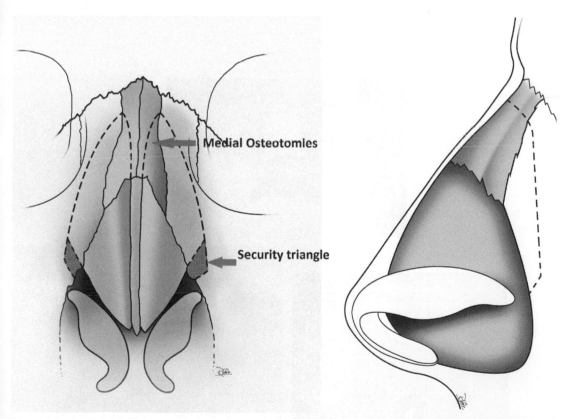

Fig. 6. Osteotomies. Medial curved ostetomies are only performed when needed. They are curved osteotomies that are angled off the midline away from the thick nasal bone. Lateral osteotomies are done using a high-low-high technique. A small triangle of bone is left intact in the lower end of the piriform aperture to avoid pos-terior collapse of the lateral nasal wall.

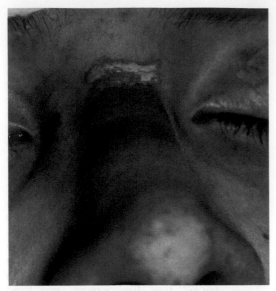

Fig. 7. Radix graft. A radix graft is usually fashioned from septal cartilage that is slightly crushed and placed in a small pocket in this area. It helps fill in a small concavity that is frequently found in Mestizo patients without having to lower the nasal dorsum.

The Middle Third of the Nose (Cartilaginous Dorsum)

The bony and cartilaginous support structures of the nose are weak in Mestizo patients. Nasal bones, as mentioned above, are short, and upper lateral cartilage (ULC) tends to be weak and collapse easily. When humps are lowered and the cartilaginous dorsum is reduced, this inherent weakness will have a natural tendency to increase, and if severe, collapse, creating important structural and functional abnormalities. It becomes important to perform preventive surgical techniques that will reinforce and, if present, correct any abnormalities in the middle cartilaginous vault.

Common anatomic findings are as follows:

a. Flattened/wide middle third of nose
b. Weak ULC
- Surgical technique: spreader grafts
   Spreader grafts are rectangular pieces of cartilage that can be carved from septal cartilage (ideal grafting material), conchal cartilage, or rib cartilage and are placed between the dorsal edge of

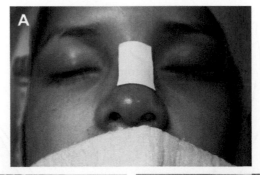

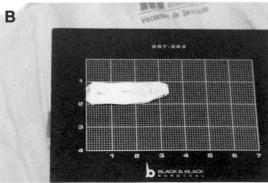

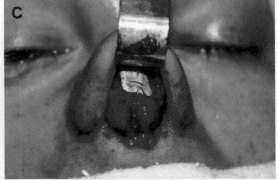

Fig. 8. Gore-Tex implants. (*A*) Gore-Tex sheeting is an alternative to augment a dorsum when cartilage is not available. (*B*) Sheets are folded and an implant is fashioned depending on patient's needs. (*C*) The implant is secured in place anteriorly with sutures to avoid postsurgical shifting.

the ULC and the nasal septum. Spreader grafts can be unilateral, bilateral, or, when needed, doubled on one of the sides. They give additional support to the middle cartilaginous vault. Its uses are countless: in primary rhinoplasty patients they can correct weak concave ULC, help straighten a crooked dorsal septum, and widen a narrow middle third of the nose. In revision cases, they help correct inverted v deformities, nasal valve collapse, and depressions of the middle third of the nose (**Fig. 9**).

Dimensions:

Thickness: 1–3 mm
Length: 18–25 mm
Width: 3–5 mm

- Surgical techniques: mattress sutures/flaring mattress sutures

Mattress sutures using a 4-0 polidioxanon foil (PDS) or absorbable material (Vicryl) can be used to further align the ULC to the dorsal edge of the septum or to align slight dorsal deviations. Flaring sutures can be placed in the ULC to open a collapsed nasal valve or to widen slightly a narrow middle third of the nose.

- Surgical techniques: onlay grafts

These grafts can be used to fill in and hide any irregularities seen in the middle cartilaginous septum. Grafts can be morcelized or edges beveled so they will not be noticeable over time. When possible, these grafts should be fixed in place so they will not shift over time.

Lower Third of the Nose (Nasal Tip)

The lower third of the nose, also known as the nasal tip, is formed by 2 important structures: the

pedestal and the nasal tripod. The pedestal is a more rigid structure formed by the nasal spine and the caudal end of the septum. The nasal tripod sits on top of the pedestal and is a flexible structure formed by the conjoined medial crura and both lateral crura. The combination of these 2 structures, with its covering, the S-STE, gives the final shape to the nasal tip. The pedestal should be structured and aligned before any important tip work is done. In this way, changes that are done on the tip will not be lost because of lack of support.[9]

The pedestal

The cartilaginous septum in Mestizo patients tends to be modest with a thickness that can vary between 2 and 3 mm. Frequently, naturally short and retrusive caudal septums can be found, which result in an acute nasolabial angle and a short columella.

Common anatomic findings are as follows:

- Small nasal spine, normal caudal septum, flimsy medial crura
- Surgical technique: columellar strut

The easiest way to structure a pedestal that needs some support is using a columellar strut. The ideal grafting material is the cartilaginous septum because it is a stronger piece of cartilage but conchal cartilage can also be used with good results. A small pocket is created between the medial crura, and the graft is sutured in place with 5-0 absorbable Vicryl sutures. It is important that the graft does not go all the way down to the nasal spine and that it does not touch the caudal end of the septum as this can produce an uncomfortable clicking sensation when patients rub their nasal tips (**Fig. 10**). Fixation sutures should be placed in the middle third of the medial

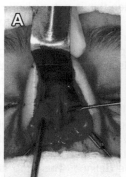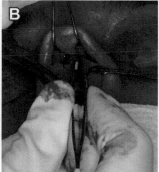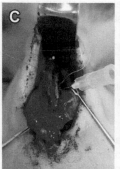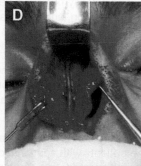

Fig. 9. Spreader grafts. (*A*) Grafts are placed in a pocket created between the dorsal edge of the septal cartilage and the ULC. (*B*) Placement of spreader graft. (*C*) The spreader graft is fixed with a 30-gauge needle and sutured in place. (*D*) Bilateral spreader grafts sutured in place. Dorsal edge of septum should be at the same level of the spreader grafts.

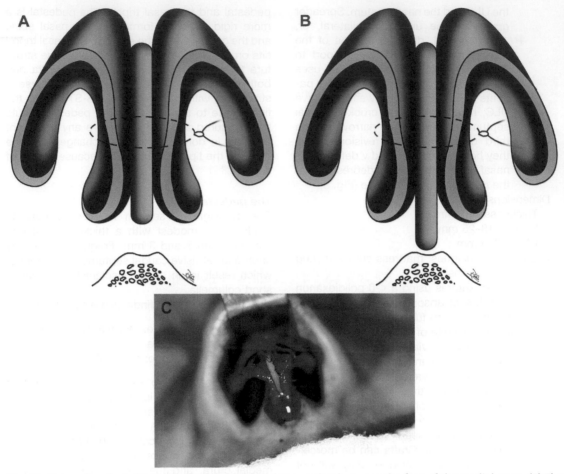

Fig. 10. Columellar strut. (*A*) Columellar strut is placed in a pocket between the feet of the medial crura. (*B*) The columellar strut ideally should not go all the way down to the nasal spine unless it is securely fixed in place to avoid shifting to the sides of the septum. (*C*) Surgical image of strut fixed in place.

crura, taking care not to place them near the dome area because this can efface the natural double break of the columella. The columellar strut will give additional support to the medial crura, correcting any asymmetries, helping maintain rotation and projection, and giving support to the pedestal by creating a stable base to be able to use sutures and grafts in the nasal tip (**Fig. 11**).

- Small nasal spine, short and weak caudal septum, acute nasolabial angle
- Surgical technique: caudal septal extension graft

The indications for using a septal extension graft are patients with acute nasolabial angles, severely underprojected tips, and retrusive caudal nasal septums with an inadequate ala-columellar relationship.[10] This type of graft is valuable in Mestizo patients when the columellar strut is not enough to correct a severely acute nasolabial angle or will not

give the necessary support to the pedestal. Because this is a replacement graft, the cartilage needed should have some strength and should be as straight as possible. The ideal grafting material is septal cartilage. When this is not available, conchal cartilage can be used, making sure to straighten it with sutures.

The graft is positioned posteriorly, overlapping the caudal edge of the existing nasal septum and inferiorly sitting on top of the nasal spine. These 2 positions are anchored securely in place with 4-0 absorbable sutures. The overlapping piece of cartilage should be thinned especially at the level of the nasal valve to avoid postsurgical nasal obstruction. Once the graft is secured, the position of the nasal tip should be defined. This step is done by suturing the feet of the medial crura to the caudal edge of the graft, depending on how much rotation and projection are needed. The shape of the extension graft can also be tailored

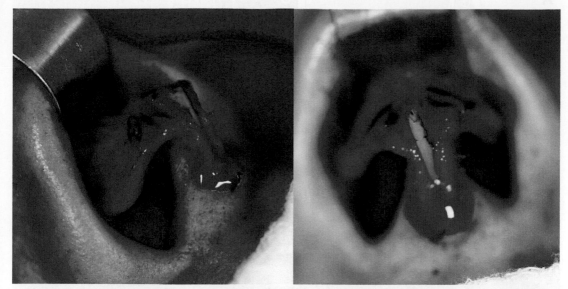

Fig. 11. Surgical image of columellar strut in place. The natural double break of the columella should be preserved when placing fixation sutures.

depending on the patient's individual needs. Although the graft usually has a rectangular shape, it can be carved wider in the inferior portion to help push out the nasolabial angle and increase rotation even more (**Fig. 12**, Video 1).

The nasal tip

Once the pedestal has been strengthened, work can safely be performed on the nasal tip. Mestizo patients want noses that look more defined; the issue is that these are usually patients that would normally require a great deal of grafting because their support structures are very poor. It becomes very important to use techniques that give support and create definition without making the nose look bigger; this is the real challenge. The common problems found in Mestizo nasal tips are as follows:

- Bulbous undefined nasal tips
- Wide flimsy alar cartilages
- Short columellas
- Poor projection and rotation

For more than 20 years, the author has been using a "gradual approach to the Mestizo tip." Alar cartilages are evaluated in their vertical and horizontal components (**Fig. 13**). The vertical component relates to how wide the cartilage is (A, B), and if it is concave or convex. The horizontal component defines the length of the alar cartilage, the width of the domal angle, and the definition of the dome (C, D).

The philosophy behind this approach is to resect very little tissue, reinforcing support structures of the nose with structural grafts when needed, and using sutures and grafts to give contour and definition to the alar cartilages. Conservative and predictable procedures are the initial surgical options, leaving the more aggressive techniques that give less predictable results to those noses with more important deformities. Suturing techniques are performed with 5-0 nonabsorbable sutures or 5-0 PDS.[11]

The surgical techniques are divided into techniques for the vertical and horizontal components. These procedures can be divided into complete strip procedures, incomplete strip procedures, and the use of grafts (see **Table 3**).

Intact tip procedures

Intact tip procedures are procedures wherein the whole strip of alar cartilage is left intact. The length of the cartilage is not changed. What can be modified is the width of the alar cartilage or the shape.

Reduction of the width of the alar cartilage

Cephalic resection of alar cartilages Cephalic trim is not done routinely by the author. Excessively wide cartilages (caudal to cephalic) can be managed with a conservative cephalic trim, leaving at least 9 to 10 mm at the lateral crus and 5 to 7 mm in the dome area. The resection should not be extended all the way into the lateral portion of the lateral crus, because this can result in supralar pinching, especially in patients with thin, flimsy cartilages.

Lateral crural turn-in-flap of cephalic portion of alar cartilage The cephalic trim is constantly replaced by the lateral crural turn-in flap. It is very useful in patients with wide and flimsy alar

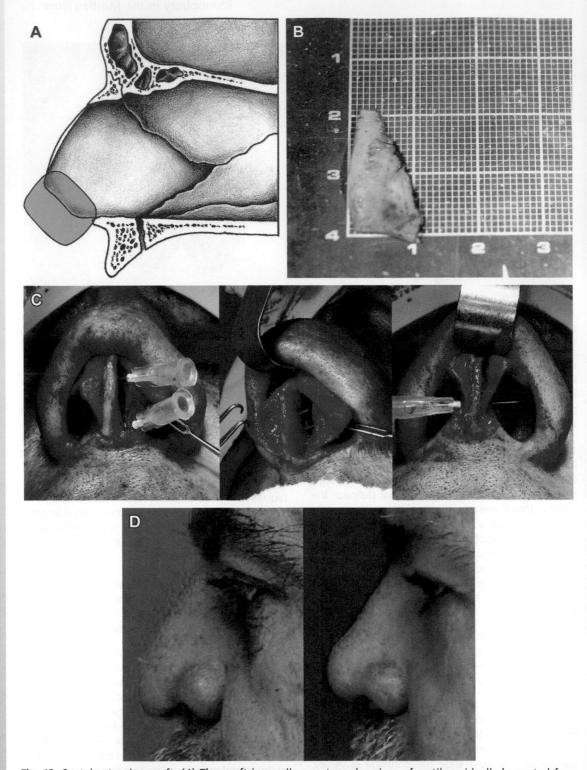

Fig. 12. Septal extension graft. (*A*) The graft is usually a rectangular piece of cartilage ideally harvested from septum. It is placed overlapping the caudal edge of the septum. (*B*) Carved piece of septal cartilage where the inferior portion is wider than the superior portion. This wide portion will be placed inferiorly over the nasal spine. (*C*) Sequence of images where the graft is fixed in a desired position with needles and sutured in place with Vicryl sutures. The inferior edge of the graft is wider than the superior edge and helps correct an overly acute nasolabial angle. (*right*) Feet of medial crura fixed in place on each side of the caudal edge of the graft with needles establishing adequate tip position. (*D*) Presurgical and 5-year postsurgical image of patient with septal extension graft.

A
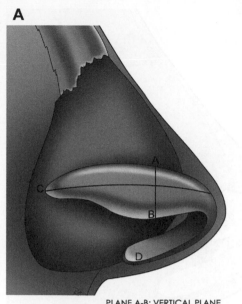

PLANE A–B: VERTICAL PLANE
PLANE C–D: HORIZONTAL PLANE

B
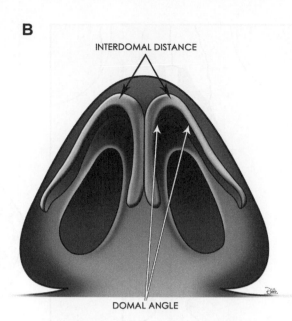

Fig. 13. Configuration of alar cartilages. (*A*) Alar cartilages have a vertical and a horizontal component. Vertically (distance A–B), this means how wide the cartilage is and evaluates if it is concave or convex. (*B*) The horizontal plane tells how long the cartilage is (distance C–D). It also gives us information on the interdomal distance and the domal angle.

cartilages. Instead of performing a cephalic resection, the portion that was going to be resected is folded on itself under the cephalic edge and sutured in place, which helps strengthen this area and improves postsurgical supralar pinching (**Fig. 14**).

Suturing techniques Suturing techniques are the first and most reliable techniques in dealing with bulbous, undefined tips. Most techniques are used to refine, project, and rotate the nasal tip. The biggest advantage they have is that if the result is not satisfactory to the surgeon, things can be easily undone until the desired result is obtained. Sutures used are 5-0 PDS or 5-0 nonabsorbable sutures. The list of possible sutures can be extremely long; only those most frequently used will be mentioned in later discussion.

Lateral crural steal Lateral crural steal is the workhorse suture used by the author with Mestizo patients.

Lateral crural steal uses include increases rotation and projection. Lateral crural steal also helps define the nasal tip by creating a more triangular-looking nasal base.

In the lateral crural steal technique, the existing dome is marked and the place where the new dome is going to be placed is also marked. This spot is usually 3- to 5-mm lateral to the existing dome. The vestibular skin is dissected from the

undersurface of the working area. Rotation is achieved by lengthening the medial crura and shortening the lateral crura (**Fig. 15**).[12]

Dome-defining sutures Uses for the dome-defining sutures include increasing the definition and projection of the nasal tip.

The technique for dome-defining sutures is a simple mattress suture that is placed at the level of the dome to narrow the dome area. When the alar cartilage is very thin, it is not uncommon to see a small concavity form after the suture is tied. In these cases, a small cartilage graft can be placed to fill in this defect and in this way avoid postsurgical pinching (**Fig. 16**).

Alar spanning suture Alar spanning suture corrects bulbosity and can increase rotation slightly.

Alar spanning suture is a mattress suture that is placed directly behind the domes in the cephalic margin of the alar cartilages and is tied in the midline. This technique narrows a wide nasal tip and helps correct excessive width without having to perform resections.[13]

Septocolumellar suture Septocolumellar suture maintains and can slightly increase projection and rotation.

The septocolumellar suture technique is a single loop suture usually done with 5-0 nonabsorbable material that is introduced from a point low at the

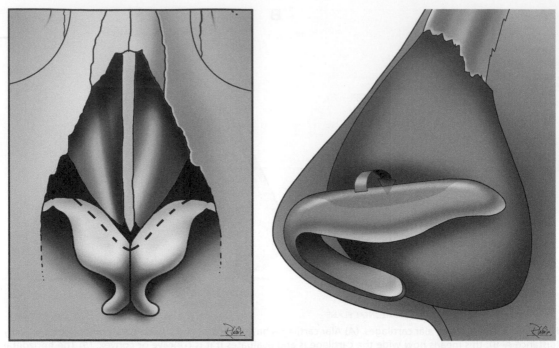

Fig. 14. Lateral crural turn-in flap. The lateral crural turn-in flap is an excellent alternative to the cephalic trim. The cephalic portion of the lateral crura is folded on itself, sutured in place, and helps prevent supralar pinching in thin flimsy alar cartilages. An *arrow* shows how the cephalic edge of the cartilage is folded inwards.

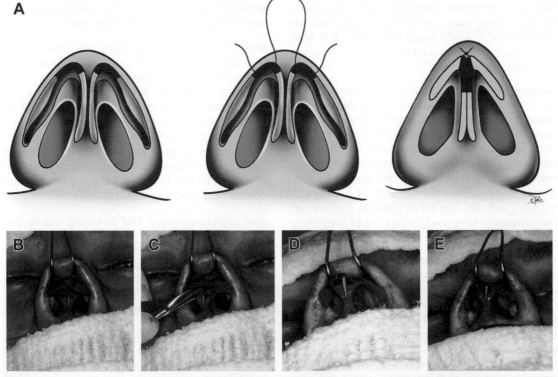

Fig. 15. Lateral crural steal. (*A*) Schematic drawing showing how tip can be rotated and projected by increasing length of medial crura at the expense of the lateral crura. (*B*) Marking of original dome and new dome. (*C*) Dissection of underlying mucosa. (*D*) Placement of new domal suture. Right dome height is increased. (*E*) Lateral crural steal is completed. Tip projection has gained projection and rotation.

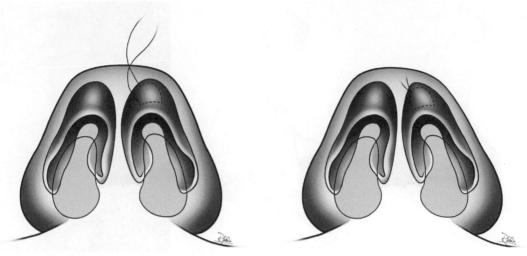

Fig. 16. Dome-defining suture. When the domal area is wide and undefined, a mattress suture can be placed to narrow the dome and help define the area. Sutures should not be overly tightened as this can result in a "pinched-looking" nasal tip.

feet of the medial crura on one side, is passed at a point near the dorsal edge of the caudal septum, and taken out at the opposite side at the foot of the medial crura of that side. The knot is tied in the midline, bringing the medial crura/columellar complex close to the caudal septum. It is imperative to have a stable pedestal that is in the midline so the whole nasal tip will not shift to one side (**Fig. 17**).

Incomplete strip procedures

Alar cartilages should be divided in those patients with an overprojecting nose or a long plunging tip. The techniques commonly used by the author are the lateral crural overlay and/or the medial crural overlay techniques. With these procedures, the alar strip is incised but is again reconstructed by overlapping the incised fragments. In this way, the alar strip is shortened without losing its support.[11,12]

Lateral crural overlay The lateral crural overlay uses long plunging nasal tips, where the lateral crura are much longer than the medial crura. The final result is shortening of the lateral crura with rotation of the nasal tip and shortening of the nose.

An incision is placed on the alar cartilage 10-mm lateral to the defined dome. The proximal and distal segments are elevated free from the underlying mucosa and the medial segment is superimposed over the lateral segment and sutured firmly in place. How much is superimposed will depend on how much rotation is wanted and how much the nose will be shortened. It usually varies from 3 to 5 mm (**Fig. 18**).

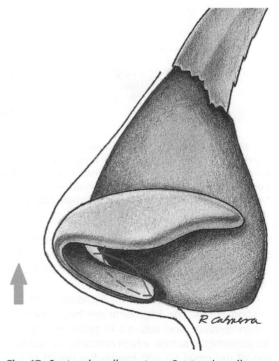

Fig. 17. Septocolumellar suture. Septocolumellar suture is a single-loop permanent suture that is placed starting at the feet of the medial crura going up toward the anterior septal angle at its dorsal edge and coming down to the feet of the medial crura of the opposite side. This pushes up the entire crura/strut complex against the caudal edge of the septum, elevating the nasal tip. An *arrow* shows how the columelar-strut complex is slightly pushed upwards.

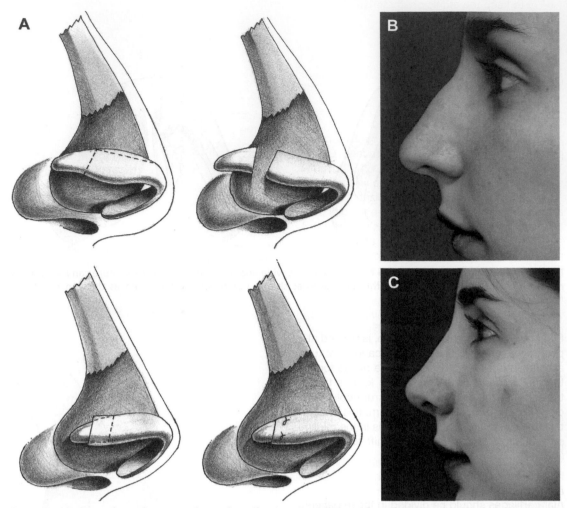

Fig. 18. Lateral crural overlay. Lateral crural overlay is an excellent technique indicated in long plunging tips where the lateral crura are overly long. (*A*) The domes are marked and an incision is placed 10-mm lateral to the dome area. The proximal and distal flaps are elevated, overlapped, and sutured in place. How much of overlapping is done will depend on how much rotation and deprojection of the nose is needed. (*B, C*) Presurgical and 7-year postsurgical image of patient where lateral crural overlay technique was used.

Medial crural overlay Medial crural overlay is often used in patients with asymmetric medial crura or long noses that have long medial and lateral crura.

An incision is placed a few millimeters below the existing dome. The fragments are then elevated, superimposed, and sutured in place with a 5-0 nonabsorbable suture, which creates counterrotation of the nasal tip and lowers the height of the dome (**Fig. 19**).

Grafts

Grafts are pieces of cartilage taken from the nasal septum, the auricular concha, or the rib cartilage that are used to give support (structural grafts), to define structures, to fill in defects, or as camouflage. Mestizo patients have noses with poor support and definition. Because the amount of cartilage is limited, it is important to plan carefully and decide wisely where the cartilage is going to be used. Whenever possible, grafts should be sutured in place especially in the nasal tip to avoid postsurgical shifting.

Shield graft A shield graft helps improve definition of the nasal tip. It can increase projection and can lengthen the tip slightly.

Ideally a shield graft should be carved from septal cartilage, although conchal cartilage and rib cartilage can be used with good results. The graft should be carved according to the specific patient's needs, but measurements can vary from 8 to 12 mm on the leading edge, 8 to

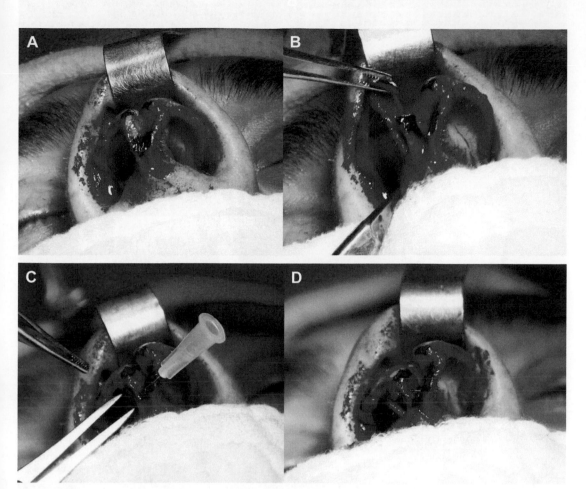

Fig. 19. Medial crural overlay. This technique is used to deproject and counterrotate the nasal tip. (*A, B*) Incision is placed a few millimeters below the existing dome. Flaps are elevated. (*C, D*) Fragments are overlapped and sutured in place. Dome is lowered on the right side.

15 mm in length, and 1 to 3 mm in thickness. The graft is sutured to the caudal margins of the medial/intermediate crural complex with 6-0 nonabsorbable sutures. The leading edge of the graft should be carved at the level of the domes and in thick-skinned patients a few millimeters above the domes. The leading edge should be well beveled and covered with morcelized cartilage or perichondrium so it will not be visible over time (**Fig. 20**).

Alar strut grafts Alar strut grafts are structural grafts that give additional support to flimsy lateral crura and that will help flatten a convex or concave lateral crus.

A thin rectangular piece of cartilage is placed in the undersurface of the lateral crus of the alar cartilage and fixed in place with absorbable sutures. The edge of the graft should not distort the dome area (**Fig. 21**A).

Alar rim grafts Alar rim grafts are structural grafts that correct flaring, correct contour irregularities, and give additional support to ala to prevent collapse of lateral sidewall.

Alar rim grafts are thin, long pieces of cartilage that are placed along the alar rim in a nonanatomic position. The superior edge of the graft should not extend all the way up to the soft tissue triangle because it can produce asymmetries in this area. The superior leading edge of the graft should be crushed gently so it will not become noticeable over time (see **Fig. 21**B).

Morcelized cartilage/crushed cartilage Crushed cartilage is frequently used to fill in small defects. Morcelized cartilage has more texture, is pliable, and can be manipulated as a single unit. It is ideal to smooth out irregularities and soften sharp edges. They are frequently used in the nasal tip and supratip area.

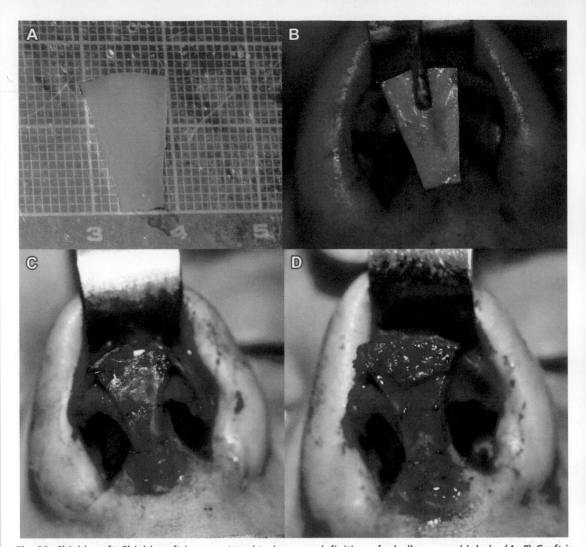

Fig. 20. Shield graft. Shield graft is a great tool to improve definition of a bulbous nasal lobule. (*A, B*) Graft is carved ideally from septal cartilage and placed in front of the medial crura/strut complex. (*C, D*) Graft is sutured in place with 6-0 nonabsorbable sutures, leaving the wide superior leading edge at the level or slightly above the domes. The leading edge ideally should be covered with morcelized cartilage to avoid visibility over time.

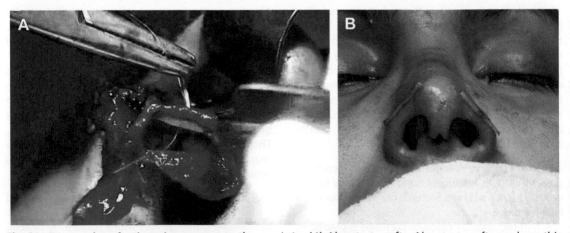

Fig. 21. Structural grafts that give support to the nasal tip. (*A*) Alar strut grafts. Alar strut grafts are long thin rectangular pieces of cartilage that are placed in the undersurface of the existing lateral crura of the alar cartilage. They strengthen the cartilage and correct concavities or convexities. (*B*) Alar rim grafts. Alar rim grafts are long thin pieces of cartilage placed in the alar rim caudal to the caudal margin of the alar cartilage. They help correct alar flaring and give additional strength to the alar rim.

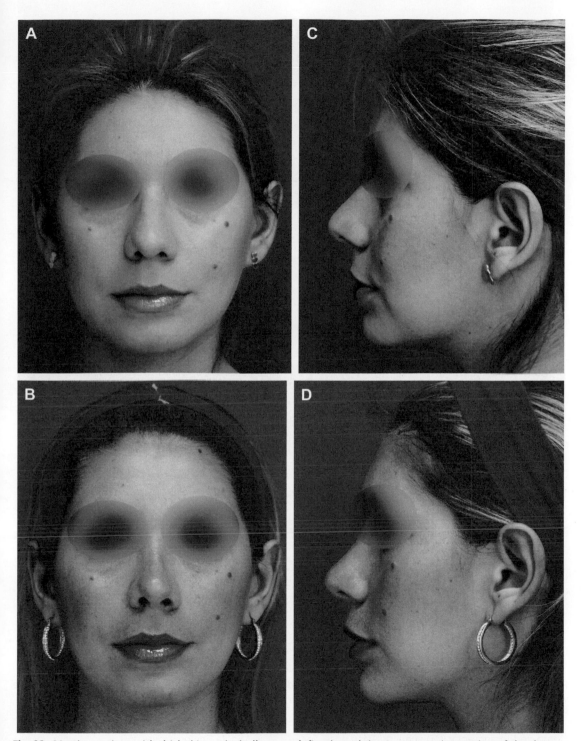

Fig. 22. Mestizo patient with thick skin and a bulbous undefined nasal tip. A conservative rasping of the dorsum was performed with placement of morcelized cartilage in the radix. The middle third of the nose was strengthened by placing bilateral spreader grafts. Lateral osteotomies were performed. The medial crura were supported with a columellar strut. Definition of the nasal tip was achieved by performing a lateral crural steal with dome-defining sutures and a lateral crural spanning suture. The cephalic margin of the alar cartilages was not trimmed; instead, a lateral crural turn-in-flap was performed. A piece of morcelized cartilage was placed over the new tip structure to help hide irregularities and alar rim grafts were placed to give additional support to the lateral ala.

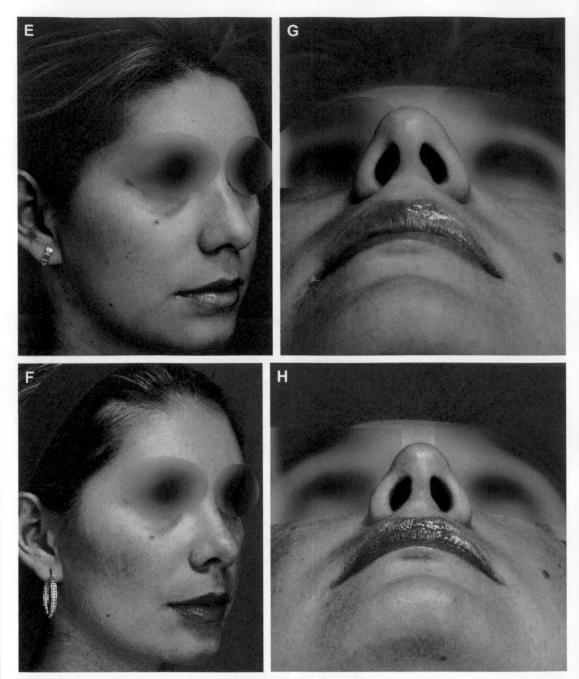

Fig. 22. (*continued*). Mestizo patient with thick skin and a bulbous undefined nasal tip. (*A, C, E, G*) Preoperative views. (*B, D, F, H*) 18 months postoperative views.

Any type of cartilage can be used but the ideal material is septal cartilage. A cartilage crusher is used and the technique is refined by trying to obtain a thin piece of cartilage that is soft and pliable and that will not break into pieces when manipulated. It should be like a carpet that can be placed as a covering over the different areas of the nose. If possible, it should be sutured in place so it will not shift over time.[11]

The Nasal Base

The alar base is evaluated after the surgery has been completed, all grafts are in place, and sutures are closed. After the desired rotation, projection, definition, and structural support to the nose have been obtained, it is not infrequent to find that the nostrils have attained a configuration that is more normal and that base reduction becomes unnecessary. When performed, it should be done because there is a need to decrease alar flare, alar base width, or both. If reduction is going to be done, incisions should be placed carefully, taking care not to extend them into the alar groove because this can leave unsightly scars especially in thick, oily, sebaceous skins.

Postsurgical Follow-up

When planning surgery, it is very important for patients to understand that an adequate postsurgical follow-up is very important. Stitches and cast are removed after 8 days and the nose is taped for an extra week. Skin care is a priority in Mestizo patients. A cleansing regimen is organized to control breakouts and acne exacerbations. Sometimes, patients need to be managed by a dermatologist. Long-term follow-up is very important and is the only objective way results can be evaluated. Post surgical photographs are taken at least 6 months and 1 year postoperatively and then on an annual or biannual basis if possible.

Case Presentation

When evaluating Mestizo patients, it is important to define what patients want and how much cartilage will be available for grafting. Postsurgical views should be taken at least after 6 months and ideally after 1 year to be able to evaluate the nose after inflammation has subsided (**Fig. 22**).

SUMMARY

Rhinoplasty is the facial plastic procedure that is more frequently performed in Mestizo patients. These noses have a poor osteocartilaginous framework and thick S-STE. A structural approach was presented where there is minimal tissue excision; structural grafts are used to strengthen and increase support structures of the nose, and using a gradual approach, sutures and grafts are used to increase rotation projection and definition of the nasal tip. Establishing a solid patient-physician relationship will definitely improve surgical outcomes. The final goal of surgery is to be able to obtain results that bring patients closer to what their cosmetic ideal is.

SUPPLEMENTARY DATA

Supplementary data related to this article can be found online at http://dx.doi.org/10.1016/j.fsc.2014.04.011.

REFERENCES

1. The Hispanic population 2010-census brief. Available at: www.census.gov.
2. Cobo R. Trends in facial plastic surgery in Latin America. Facial Plast Surg 2013;29:149–53.
3. Ospina W. América Mestiza-El país del Futuro. Bogotá (Colombia): Villegas Editores; 2000. p. 23–38.
4. Cobo R. Mestizo rhinoplasty. Facial Plast Surg 2003; 19(3):257–68.
5. Toriumi D, Johnson C. Open rhinoplasty—featured technical points and long-term follow-up. Facial Plast Surg Clin North Am 1993;1(1):1–22.
6. Becker D, Pastorek NJ. The radix graft in cosmetic rhinoplasty. Arch Facial Plast Surg 2001;3(2):115–9.
7. Romo T III, Abraham MT. The ethnic nose. Facial Plast Surg 2003;19(3):269–77.
8. Godin MS, Waldman SR, Johnson CM. Nasal augmentation using Gore-Tex. A 10-year experience. Arch Facial Plast Surg 1999;1(2):118–21.
9. Johnson CM, To WC. The tripod-pedestal concept. In: Johnson C Jr, Wyatt C, editors. A case approach to open structure rhinoplasty. 1st edition. Philadelphia: Elsevier Saunders; 2005. p. 9–20.
10. Toriumi DM. New concepts in nasal tip contouring. Arch Facial Plast Surg 2006;8(3):156–85.
11. Cobo R. Nuances with the Mestizo tip. Facial Plast Surg 2012;28:202–12.
12. Konior RJ, Kridel R. Controlled nasal tip positioning via the open rhinoplasty approach. Facial Plast Surg Clin North Am 1993;1(1):53–62.
13. Perkins S, Patel A. Endonasal suture techniques in tip rhinoplasty. Facial Plast Surg Clin North Am 2009;17:41–54.

Asian Blepharoplasty

Samuel M. Lam, MD

KEYWORDS

- Asian blepharoplasty • Supratarsal crease • Ethnic facial plastic surgery • Double eyelid
- Full-incision Asian blepharoplasty

KEY POINTS

- Maintaining a low crease height is important for a natural, ethnically sensitive outcome.
- Always work in an alternating fashion during surgery to increase the chances for a symmetric result.
- The full-incision method has a higher likelihood of a long-term, tenacious crease result than more abbreviated incision approaches.

INTRODUCTION

Asian blepharoplasty is defined as the surgical creation of a supratarsal crease in an individual who has either a partial presence of a fold or an entire absence of it.[1-4] There are many methods and variations to create a supratarsal crease in someone who was born without one, including the full-incision, partial-incision, and no-incision methods. Having studied and performed all three major methods, I have found that the full-incision method offers the most durable crease fixation, wider surgical exposure, precise ability to attain a defined crease shape, and can favorably modulate dermatochalasis associated with aging. However, the principal trade off is a significantly more protracted recovery period associated with the longer incision. Interestingly, scarring is less obvious in my opinion with the full-incision method compared with the partial-incision technique because the abrupt ends of the partial incision terminate in the middle of the eyelid and can be relatively more conspicuous.

This article details the full-incision method that has served me well over the past decade in practice so that the reader grasps the requisite preoperative, intraoperative, and postoperative considerations for the Asian patient desiring an upper-eyelid crease. The focus of this article centers on the younger Asian patient (<40 years old)

who simply would like to create a supratarsal crease. Management of the aging Asian eyelid is a more complicated subject, and I have written about my strategy elsewhere in the literature.

TREATMENT GOALS AND PLANNED OUTCOME

First, it is worth reviewing some fundamental and relevant anatomy that pertains to the Asian eyelid. In the Occidental eyelid (and in some Asians), the levator aponeurosis inserts into the dermis to create the natural supratarsal crease (**Fig. 1**). In the Asian there is a partial adhesion or an entire absence of the adhesion leading to variable degrees of crease presence. In addition, what leads to the narrower palpebral fissure (eye opening) and fuller, puffy eyelid appearance is the presence of orbital fat that descends lower toward the ciliary margin because the levator muscle does not prohibit its descent. Accordingly, in many cases I do not remove much fat (unless the fat is excessive and prohibits a strong levator-to-skin adhesion). Also, I have a proclivity to preserve fat because I am a proponent of fat grafting to restore lost volume related to aging, so I would not want to accelerate perceived aging through overzealous fat removal.

Culturally, it is worth discussing the evolution of an aesthetic over the past 30 plus years. In the

Disclosures: None.
Willow Bend Wellness Center, 6101 Chapel Hill Boulevard, Suite 101, Plano, TX 75093, USA
E-mail address: drlam@lamfacialplastics.com

Facial Plast Surg Clin N Am 22 (2014) 417–425
http://dx.doi.org/10.1016/j.fsc.2014.04.002

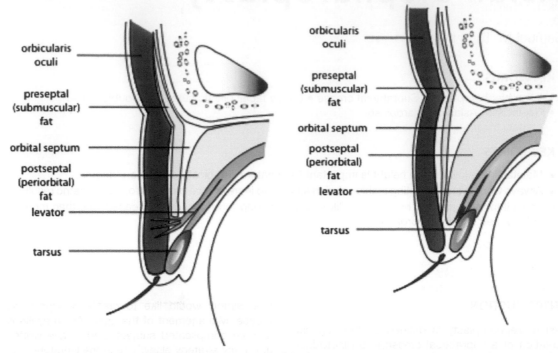

Fig. 1. The occidental eyelid (*left*) shows the insertion of the levator aponeurosis into the dermis that creates the natural crease of the western eyelid. In the Asian eyelid (*right*), the levator does not insert into the skin, so there is no crease. In addition, the postseptal fat can slide down more toward the ciliary margin making the palpebral aperture appear much smaller in size. (*From* Lam SM. Asian blepharoplasty. In: McCurdy JA, Lam SM, editors. Cosmetic surgery of the Asian face. 2nd edition. New York: Thieme Medical Publishers; 2005. p. 10; with permission.)

1980s, the term "Westernization" was highly popular, because many Asians truly wanted to look white, but this surgery involved excessive fat and skin removal along with a very high crease fixation. This technique led to extremely artificial-looking results that did not appear white or Asian but simply alien in nature. Today, the watchword is cultural and ethnic preservation, which can subtly but dramatically enhance the appearance of an individual. Creases are low and eyelids have a much fuller configuration; those are the only types of creases that I make, because it is outside of my desire to produce results that do not live up to a high aesthetic standard of naturalness and beauty.

Besides aesthetic enhancement, other motivating factors for Asian patients may include better assimilation into a Western society, ease with applying makeup (because there is now a fold into which the eye shadow can reside), improved vision afforded by a wider palpebral aperture, and more rarely a superstition of improved good fortune based on ancient Asian folkloric beliefs. The surgeon should obviously be well informed, sensitive, and exploratory during the preoperative counseling phase to ensure a mutually satisfactory outcome for patient and surgeon alike. During the consultation, the surgeon should discuss the desired aesthetic shape and height of the supratarasal crease (discussed in the next section) along with the protracted nature of the recovery period and what can be done to ameliorate the convalescent experience (discussed in the subsequent, relevant section).

A thorough anatomic evaluation of the patient's eyelids should be undertaken and reviewed with the prospective patient. Asymmetry is perhaps one of the most commonly encountered attributes in the preoperative eyelid, and this condition most often stems from one side having a greater degree of partial fixation than the other side. The reason for this asymmetry is that the side with a greater degree of fixation typically has less of the fat descending toward the ciliary margin (as explained previously) and thereby a wider eye opening. Fortunately, this asymmetry can be greatly improved by simply making two equal surgical crease fixations. Accordingly, in most cases it is inadvisable to perform a unilateral eyelid crease because the other side will most likely not match the newly formed side.

PROCEDURAL APPROACH
Designing the Proposed Eyelid Crease

The first order of business is to confirm and elaborate on the shape and height of the eyelid crease again with the patient. There are two principles shapes, oval and round, and two principal crease configurations, open and closed (**Fig. 2**). The oval shape refers to a flared configuration in which the lateral terminus of the crease is higher than the medial side. The round shape refers to a crease height that is parallel to the ciliary margin throughout its entire extent. The inside fold refers to a crease that terminates inside (lateral) to the epicanthus, whereas an outside fold runs parallel and medial to the epicanthus. As one can imagine,

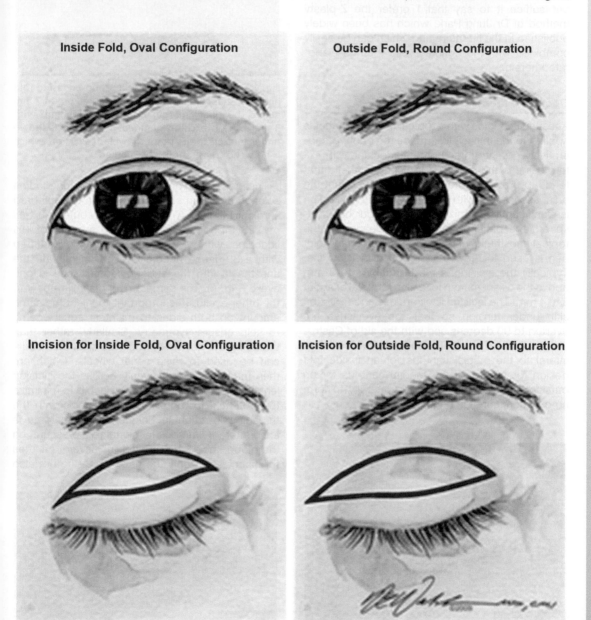

Fig. 2. There are two principles shapes, oval and round, and two principal crease configurations, open and closed. The oval shape refers to a flared configuration in which the lateral terminus of the crease is higher than the medial side. The round shape refers to a crease height that is parallel to the ciliary margin throughout its entire extent. The inside fold refers to a crease that terminates inside (lateral) to the epicanthus, whereas an outside fold runs parallel and medial to the epicanthus. (*From* Lam SM. Asian blepharoplasty. In: Larrabee WF, Gassner HG, Walsh WE, editors. The art and craft of facial rejuvenation surgery. Beijing (China): People's Medical Publishing House; 2013; with permission.)

typically an inside fold naturally pairs with an oval eyelid shape, and an outside fold works well with a round-shaped design. Personally, if the patient does not have a preference, I recommend the inside fold, oval configuration combination, because I believe it has the greatest aesthetic appeal. The methods of epicanthoplasty design, strategy, and execution lie beyond the scope of this article but suffice it to say that I prefer the Z-plasty method of Dr Jung Park, which has been widely published in the literature and which can be easily combined with the double-eyelid method elaborated herein.

Operative Steps

Anesthesia begins with a topical anesthesia that is applied to the thin eyelid surface for 1 hour preoperatively. Twenty-three percent lidocaine with 7% tetracaine is the preferred topical anesthetic that tends to provide profound anesthesia so that the pain associated with local-anesthetic infiltration is significantly minimized. After an hour has transpired, the patient's eyelids are cleaned of the topical anesthetic, and a fine-tipped gentian violet pen is used to draw the proposed incision line. Typically the incision is made about 7 to 9 mm above the ciliary margin for a skin removal of about 3 to 4 mm. The incision lines are designed with the skin under tension so that the eyelashes are everted to 90 degrees and with the aid of Castroviejo calipers (**Fig. 3**). The incision line can stop lateral to the medial canthus for an inside fold design (or medial to the medial canthus for an outside fold) and can be flared laterally to form an oval configuration (**Figs. 4** and **5**).

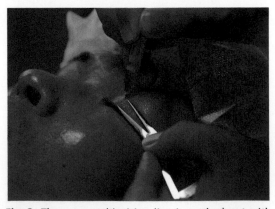

Fig. 3. The proposed incision line is marked out with the skin under tension to the point of eversion of the eyelashes to 90 degrees and with the use of Castroviejo calipers. Typically, the inferior limb of the incision is marked out at 7 to 9 mm above the ciliary margin.

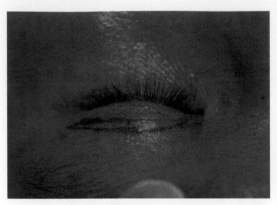

Fig. 4. This photograph shows a proposed inside fold and oval-shaped designed crease marked out at 7 mm above the ciliary margin for the inferior limb with 3 mm of skin excision planned. The eyelid is shown under tension to the point of eyelash eversion, which is how the crease should be marked.

The face is then prepared using povidone-iodine solution and then sterilely draped in the standard surgical fashion. A 1-mL syringe containing half of 0.25% bupivacaine 1:100,000 and half of 1% lidocaine with 1:100,000 epinephrine outfitted with a 30-gauge needle is used to infiltrate the anesthesia into the subcutaneous tissue in one eyelid (**Fig. 6**). The same amount is infiltrated into the other eyelid. It is important to inject the same amount on both sides to maintain equal edema to help ensure symmetry. Similarly, rather than threading the needle through the skin, the needle can be used to raise serial wheals, which are then massaged more evenly across the incision length. The reason for this approach is to minimize the potential for untoward ecchymosis with the threading injection technique. If a hematoma is encountered, immediate sustained pressure on the globe should be applied for several minutes to minimize not only the risk of bruising but also

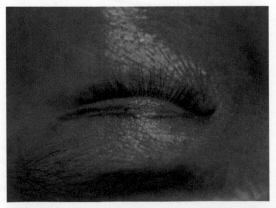

Fig. 5. This photograph shows the same as in **Fig. 4** but without the skin held under tension.

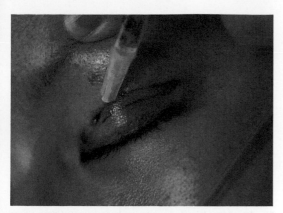

Fig. 6. This photograph shows the application of local anesthesia using a total of 1 mL per side. Specific details as to the technique are given in the text.

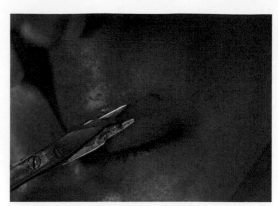

Fig. 8. A strip of remaining orbicularis oculi and preseptal tissue is removed along the inferior wound edge to debulk the pretarsal tissue and to more easily access the postseptal fat pad.

the risk of not being able to read symmetry because of the unilateral swelling. Because of the low dose of anesthesia, which minimizes intraoperative and postoperative edema that can in turn obscure the ability to read symmetry, the time that the anesthesia wears off is approximately slightly less than an hour, so the surgeon should work in an expeditious fashion to complete the operative case.

Next, a No. 15 Bard-Parker blade is used to incise through the skin but not too deeply so that the multiple, superficial vascular arcades are not transected but instead allowed to be coagulated with bipolar cautery (**Fig. 7**). A strip of remaining orbicularis oculi and preseptal tissue is removed along the inferior wound edge to debulk the pretarsal tissue and to more easily access the postseptal fat pad (**Fig. 8**). With the help of the assistant who

applies pressure above and below to push the postseptal fat forward, the surgeon makes a small fenestration laterally along the preseptal tissue until the fat herniates through the defect (**Fig. 9**). Finding the fat is the requisite step to ensure that the surgeon remains above the levator and thereby avoid injury to the underlying levator. Mosquito clamps are used to elevate the preseptal tissues upward and away from the underlying fat and levator (**Fig. 10**). Then, bipolar cautery is applied to limit bleeding (**Fig. 11**) before the preseptal tissues are widely opened with scissors (**Fig. 12**). The same technique is applied medially to the fenestration to achieve complete exposure to the postseptal tissue and the levator.

With the fat widely exposed, any excess fat can be conservatively removed with a Mosquito clamp (**Fig. 13**) after 1% lidocaine plain is infiltrated into

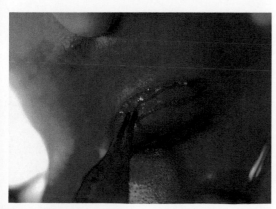

Fig. 7. This photograph shows the use of bipolar cautery to achieve hemostasis along the exposed vascular arcades that typically run perpendicular to the length of the incision immediately below the skin surface.

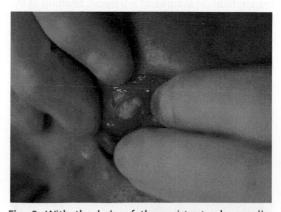

Fig. 9. With the help of the assistant who applies pressure above and below to push the postseptal fat forward, the surgeon makes a small fenestration laterally along the preseptal tissue until the fat herniates through the defect.

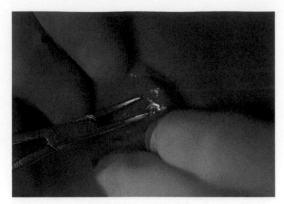

Fig. 10. Mosquito clamps are used to elevate the preseptal tissues upward and away from the underlying fat and levator.

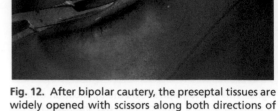

Fig. 12. After bipolar cautery, the preseptal tissues are widely opened with scissors along both directions of the initial fenestration.

the fat pad for added comfort, taking care not to allow any lidocaine to drip onto the levator, which could in turn cause levator dysfunction. In most cases, I do not remove any fat but just sweep the fat upward and away from the point of fixation. However, if there is a true exuberance of fat tissue, I remove some of the fat to minimize the puffy eyelid contour and to limit the risk that the fat will interfere with the crease fixation.

A cotton-tip applicator should be used to sweep the remaining fat away from the levator until the glistening white structure of the levator is completely in view. At times, the posterior leaf of the orbital septum, which manifests as a thin wispy layer, remains and must be swept or trimmed away to expose the levator below. With the levator fully exposed, the surgeon should now progress to the opposite eyelid and perform the same sequence of steps until both levator complexes are in full view. Now the task is to start performing crease fixation sutures of 5-0 nylon. Starting at the

midpupil, the suture is passed through the skin edge running inferiorly to superiorly (**Fig. 14**). Next, the suture is passed horizontally through the levator (**Fig. 15**). Finally, the suture is passed through the superior wound edge running inferiorly to superiorly (**Fig. 16**) and then tied down. With the patient's eyes opened the eyelashes should evert to about 90 degrees (**Fig. 17**). The crease height looks too high at this point, and that is normal. The end goal is a symmetric crease height and properly everted eyelashes (but not beyond 90 degrees).

After the first fixation suture is completed, the surgeon then performs the exact same fixation suture at the midpupil of the opposite eye. The surgeon should carefully observe the two sides for symmetry and proper eyelash eversion. If there is too much eyelash eversion and/or if the crease height is too high, then the fixation suture can be replaced slightly lower along the levator and vice

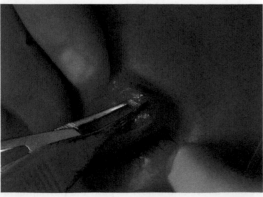

Fig. 11. Bipolar cautery is applied along both sides of the fenestration to help achieve hemostasis before the preseptal tissues are incised.

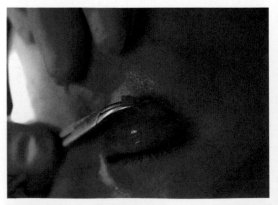

Fig. 13. With the fat exposed if there is an excess of fat, a conservative amount is removed as needed to reduce the puffy eyelid contour and to minimize the risk that the fat will obstruct the crease fixation.

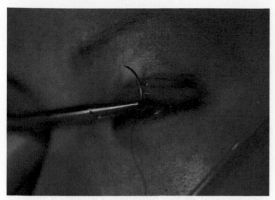

Fig. 14. Starting at the midpupil, a 5-0 nylon suture is passed through the skin edge running inferiorly to superiorly as the first of three steps in the process of creating a crease fixation.

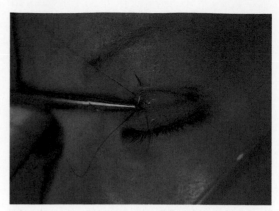

Fig. 16. Finally, the suture is passed through the superior wound edge running inferiorly to superiorly and then tied down.

versa. Additional crease fixation sutures should be applied along the entire length of the incision, typically two more crease fixation sutures medial to the midpupil suture (eg, at the medial limbus and halfway between the medial limbus and medial canthus), and two additional crease fixation sutures lateral to the original suture (eg, at the lateral limbus and halfway between the lateral limbus and lateral canthus). Additional sutures can be applied as needed. The surgeon should always work in an alternating fashion, applying a suture at the same point on each eyelid and evaluate the creases for symmetry before continuing. Once all of the crease fixation sutures are applied, the skin can be closed with a running, nonlocking 7-0 nylon suture (**Fig. 18**).

POSTPROCEDURAL CARE

After the procedure, the patient uses hydrogen peroxide to clean the incision twice daily followed

immediately by the generous application of antibiotic ointment. The patient is asked to wear glasses and to avoid contact lenses for 10 days if possible.

REHABILITATION, RECOVERY, AND FOLLOW-UP

The patient needs to understand that the eyelids can look overwhelmingly puffy and the crease, too high for weeks if not months after the procedure. However, the worst time is in the first week especially with the sutures still in place. All sutures are removed at 7 days postoperatively. I have found that applying the topical anesthetic for an hour and using Castroviejo microscissors can help significantly with patient comfort during suture removal. Regarding the delicate handling of the incision, the patient is asked to still be very gentle to the incision line for an additional week because the crease fixation must take more time to adhere as perfectly as possible.

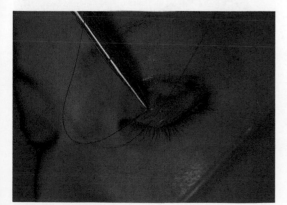

Fig. 15. Then, the same suture is passed horizontally through the levator.

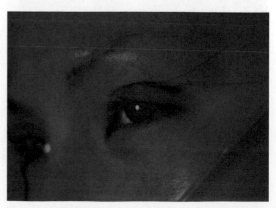

Fig. 17. With the patient's eyes opened the eyelashes should evert to about 90 degrees.

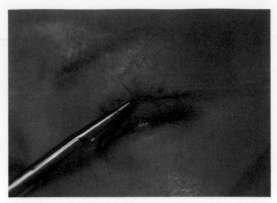

Fig. 18. A running 7-0 nylon is used to close the skin between the crease fixation sutures, with all sutures removed in 7 days postoperatively.

After the first week and after the sutures are removed, the patient starts to appear much more natural within a few days. However, the crease height still looks abnormal for several weeks to months with each successive week reducing the unsightly pretarsal edema rapidly. It can take up to a full year for complete resolution of pretarsal edema.

To help with the appearance of the eyelid edema, I recommend all my patients to wear thick framed, black rectangular glasses that sit just at the newly created supratarsal crease. This truly helps minimize the appearance of the eyelid edema. For women, I also highly recommend to start wearing eye shadow after the first 10 days to help camouflage the edema. Both of these measures truly work well.

POTENTIAL COMPLICATIONS AND MANAGEMENT

The most common complications that can occur after a full-incision Asian blepharoplasty include asymmetry, partial or complete loss of one or both folds, scarring, and an undesirable crease height and shape. For asymmetry or loss of the fold, revision surgery is mandatory to attempt improvement of the situation. Operating through a nonvirgin plane can be very difficult for even the most experienced expert in Asian blepharoplasty. As always, slow deliberate discovery of the postseptal fat laterally helps to minimize the risk of damage to the underlying levator. I typically wait 3 to 6 months before attempting revision surgery to allow for the tissues to adequately heal and with the hope that any asymmetry or abnormality in the fold dissipates as edema resolves.

OUTCOME

Like all facial cosmetic surgery procedures, the outcome of surgery should reflect the expressed taste of the surgeon and the patient alike. I have a hard time making creases that appear overly sculpted and high despite the patient's desire for

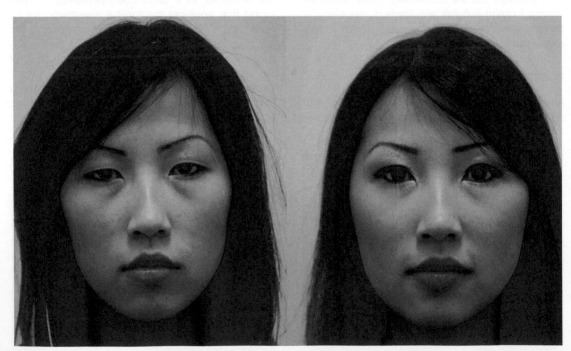

Fig. 19. This Asian patient is shown before and 1 year after supratarsal crease fixation with the design of an oval shape and inside-fold configuration.

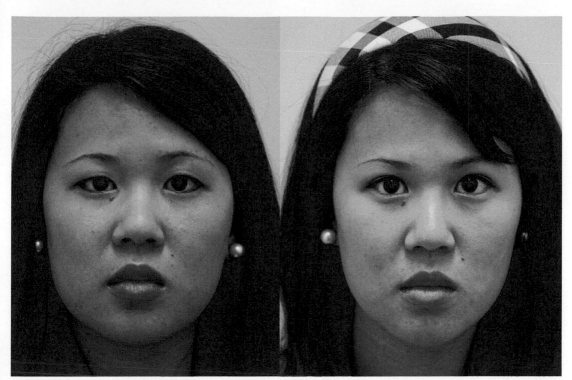

Fig. 20. This Asian patient is shown before and 1 year after supratarsal crease fixation with the design of an oval shape and inside-fold configuration.

this type of crease because it is not in alignment with my aesthetic ideals. That being said, most Asians today do not want high creases because they want to preserve their natural, ethnic appearance (**Figs. 19** and **20**).

With the stated goal of creating a supratarsal crease, the patient attains three benefits: (1) a less ethnic-appearing eyelid, (2) improved visual fields because of a more open palpebral fissure, and (3) ease of application of eyelid makeup that was impossible before surgery. If done with discretion and taste, Asian blepharoplasty can provide the patient lifelong satisfaction.

SUMMARY

Asian blepharoplasty is a technically straightforward procedure that can help a patient achieve one's desired aesthetic result. However, I believe that the procedure is not intended for the occa-

sional surgeon but one who desires to make it a worthy part of his or her surgical offering to ensure that each patient attains the best results with the minimal risk of complications.

REFERENCES

1. McCurdy JA Jr, Lam SM. Cosmetic surgery of the Asian face. 2nd edition. New York: Thieme Medical Publishers; 2005.
2. Lam SM. Aesthetic facial surgery for the Asian male. Facial Plast Surg 2005;21:317–23.
3. Lam SM. A new paradigm for the aging face. Facial Plast Surg Clin North Am 2010;18(1):1–6. Considerations in Non-Caucasian Facial Plastic Surgery.
4. Lam SM, Karam AM. Management of the Asian upper eyelid. Facial Plast Surg Clin North Am 2010;18(3): 419–26. Periocular Rejuvenation.

Fig 20. This Asian patient is shown before and 1 year after supratarsal crease fixation with the design of an oval shape and inside-fold configuration.

this type of crease because it is not in alignment with my aesthetic ideals. That being said, most Asians today do not want high creases because they want to preserve their natural, ethnic appearance (Figs 19 and 20).

With the stated goal of creating a supratarsal crease, the patient attains three benefits: (1) a less ethnic-appearing eyelid, (2) improved visual fields because of a more open palpebral fissure, and (3) ease of application of eyelid makeup that was impossible before surgery. If done with discretion and taste, Asian blepharoplasty can provide the patient lifelong satisfaction.

SUMMARY

Asian blepharoplasty is a technically straightforward procedure that can help a patient achieve one's desired aesthetic result. However, I believe that the procedure is not intended for the occa-sional surgeon but one who desires to make it a worthy part of his or her surgical offering to ensure that each patient attains the best results with the minimal risk of complications.

REFERENCES

1. McCurdy JA Jr, Lam SM. Cosmetic surgery of the Asian face. 2nd edition. New York: Thieme Medical Publishers; 2005.
2. Lam SM. Aesthetic strategies for the Asian male. Facial Plast Surg 2005;21:317-20.
3. Lam SM. A new paradigm to the aging face. Facial Plast Surg Clin North Am 2011;
   Considerations in Non-Caucasian Facial Plastic Surgery.
4. Lam SM, Karam AM. Management of the Asian upper eyelid. Facial Plast Surg Clin North Am 2010;18(1):
   418-26. Periocular Rejuvenation.

Ethnic Considerations in Hair Restoration Surgery

Jeffrey Epstein, MD[a,b,c],*, Anthony Bared, MD[b], Gorana Kuka, MD[d]

KEYWORDS

- Hair transplant • Follicular unit extraction • Ethnic hair transplant • Eyebrow transplantation
- Hispanic hair transplant • Asian hair

KEY POINTS

- Different ethnic groups have specific characteristics of the hair that affects the results of hair transplants.
- Asian hair, typically of thick caliber and dark, is often more challenging to achieve natural appearing results.
- Patients of African ethnicity are good candidates for eyebrow and scalp hair transplants, because the curly hair and minimal color contrast between scalp and hair facilitate achieving results that appear natural.
- Follicular unit extraction is the preferred technique for harvesting grafts in patients of African and most of Asian ethnicity.

INTRODUCTION

Consistent with the trends acknowledged by the other contributors in this issue of *Clinics*, and confirmed by demographic shifts in the United States, the ethnic patient constitutes a growing trend in the use of plastic surgery, and the specialty of surgical hair restoration is no exception. In our practice, with offices located in 2 ethnically diverse cities, most of our patients are non-European/nonwhite. This diversity is further magnified by the wide scope geographically in which our patients reside; more than 70% of them travel for surgery commonly from throughout Latin America but also the Middle East and Asia, including East Indians and Asians. This ethnic diversity provided to us by our international presence is duplicated by the ethnic makeup of our patients, who come from throughout North America, not only Miami and New York. In particular, this North American trend includes increasing

numbers of African Americans and also Middle Easterners, Asians, East Indians, and, of course, Hispanics seeking out hair restoration.

As hair restoration surgeons, we essentially perform 1 common procedure: hair grafting, in which hair is transplanted from the back or sides of the head into areas of hair loss, most commonly the frontal and midscalp and crown regions, but sometimes, into other areas, including the beard and eyebrows. In addition to these hair transplants, we perform several other procedures, including hairline lowering surgery (surgical hairline advancement [SHA]), in which the hairline is advanced and the forehead shortened, and the repair of previous plastic surgery procedures, including but not limited to the repair of alopecic scarring and hairline distortion caused by previous browlifts and facelifts. With these procedures, ethnic considerations affect not only technique and patient candidacy but more subtly and just

The authors have no disclosures to make.
[a] Department of Otolaryngology, University of Miami College of Medicine, University of Miami Hospital & Clinics, P.O. Box 016960 (D-48), Miami, FL 33136, USA; [b] Foundation for Hair Restoration, 6280 Sunset Drive, Suite 504, Miami, FL 33143, USA; [c] Foundation for Hair Restoration, 20 East 56th Street, 3rd Floor, New York City, NY 10021, USA; [d] Colic Hospital, Surdulička 5, Belgrade 11000, Serbia
* Corresponding author. 6280 Sunset Drive, Suite 504, Miami, FL 33143.
E-mail address: jse@drjeffreyepstein.com

Facial Plast Surg Clin N Am 22 (2014) 427–437
http://dx.doi.org/10.1016/j.fsc.2014.04.007
1064-7406/14/$ – see front matter © 2014 Elsevier Inc. All rights reserved.

as importantly, patient motives, expectations, and concepts of beauty as a result of ethnicity (ie, Middle Eastern men desiring full beards so as to appear masculine). In this article, these considerations are presented.

ANATOMIC AND HAIR CHARACTERISTIC ETHNIC DIFFERENCES

Although there exist a multitude of hair types in the lay literature, within the medical literature, human hair has been categorized into 3 ethnic groups according to distinguishable characteristics: Asian, white, and African hair. These ethnic groupings show distinct characteristics in hair density, diameter, shape, mechanical properties, and composition.[1] The hair follicle itself determines the appearance of the hair. The typical hair follicle of Asian hair is round, whereas those of whites and African are ovoid and elliptical, respectively.[2] The shape of the hair follicle is thus believed to contribute to the appearance and the geometry of the hair. Asian hair has a circular geometry, African hair has an elliptical shape, and hair of whites is of an intermediate shape. The chemical and protein composition of hair does not vary across ethnic groups, and there is no difference in the keratin types. However, African hair generally has less tensile strength and breaks more easily than hair of whites. The hair follicles of Asians are metabolically more active than those of whites, and therefore, the grafts of Asians are more vulnerable to dehydration and a prolonged preservation period.

An important issue when considering ethnic characteristics in evaluating patients for hair transplantation is the density of hairs in the donor site. This density is a product of 2 factors: the concentration of hairs and the size or caliber of each individual hair. The concentration of hairs is presented in the form of follicular units per cm^2; a single follicular unit is the natural occurring grouping of hairs as they grow in the scalp. A follicular unit, as described by Headington,[3] Sperling,[4] and Kim,[5] consists of 1 to 4 hairs, surrounding by an adventitial sheath, which also contains some supportive structures. A hair graft typically consists of a single follicular unit, which is the building block of aesthetic hair restoration. Asian hair has the largest cross-sectional diameter or caliber, whereas the density of hair is intermediate in whites (whose highest density of hair follicles is 100 follicular units/cm^2) and lowest in Africans. This characteristic may be deceptive to the novice hair transplant surgeon, because African hair gives the appearance of a higher density, given the curly nature of the hair. This characteristic is beneficial

to the patient because the appearance of higher density may be achieved with lower graft density in the recipient area. Asians have a high proportion of single hairs (24%–30% compared with 14% found in whites).

HAIR GRAFTING TO THE SCALP
Donor Site Follicle Extraction

We use 2 hair transplantation techniques: the follicular unit grafting (FUG) or strip technique and the follicular unit extraction (FUE) technique. Both use the same basic concept of transplanting hair from more permanent donor areas (usually the sides and back of the scalp, but in cases of severe limited supply of donor hairs, usually as a result of previous procedures, the donor area can be the chest or beard) into the recipient areas, where more hair is desired. FUG and FUE differ in how these donor hairs are obtained. FUG is the traditional technique of donor hair harvesting, whereby parallel incisions are made in the donor scalp area to remove a strip. The length and width of the excision depend on the amount of grafts being transplanted in the procedure. From this strip, individual FUGs are then dissected under the microscope, a process that requires a team of trained assistants, and separated out based on the number of hairs per graft (1, 2, 3, or 4).

In the FUE technique, individual punches, typically ranging in size from 0.8 to 1.0 mm, are used to extract individual follicular units from the permanent donor areas. As the fastest growing component of our practice, the FUE technique is relevant in ethnic hair transplantation cases. We perform FUE procedures almost exclusively in patients of African American and Asian ethnicity. FUE obviates the linear scar from a traditional FUG strip procedure (**Fig. 1**). Because of the geometry of the hair in Asians, resulting in more a more spiky pattern of hair growth, whereby the hairs tend to grow less vertically downward instead of growing more outward or horizontally, the linear scar in patients of Asian ethnicity can be more conspicuous. Similarly, in the African American patient, FUE provides a cosmetic advantage, because the African American patient can continue to cut his hair very short and avoid the appearance of a linear scar. The hair transplant surgeon needs to be aware of the geometry of the African American hair follicle when performing an FUE procedure. The curliness of the hair does not stop at the skin, so the surgeon needs to be cognizant of the potential change in hair direction underneath the epidermis.

In our practice, most of our FUEs are performed by a specially designed handheld drill and do not

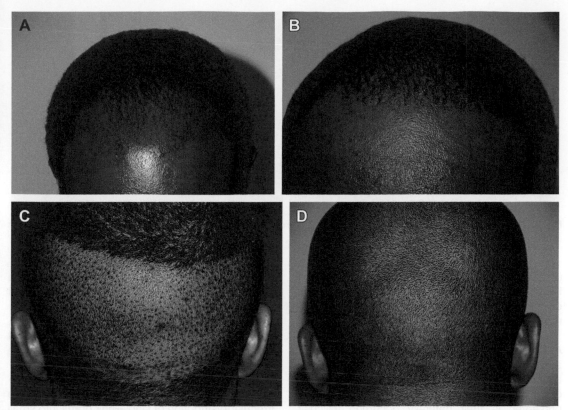

Fig. 1. FUE procedure on an African man. (*A*) Before; (*B*) 1 year after; (*C*) donor site 1 day after; (*D*) donor site 1 year after.

rely on automated extraction tools or robotic devices. We find that extracting the follicles in this way allows for minimal graft transection, even when using smaller punch sizes, which have as an advantage the reduction in scarring of the donor area. In the case of African American curly hair, blunt dissection is critical to avoid excessive graft transection. The remainder of the graft extraction then may be facilitated by forceps extraction. Hair follicles of Asians are not only straight but also tend to be longer than those of whites, and therefore, the probability of transection during FUE is higher. We suggest using a sharp punch when dissection is limited to the dermal layer (dermal papilla is on average 5–6 mm from the skin surface in Asians compared with 4–5 mm in whites), and the rest of the extraction is facilitated by forceps as well. Postoperatively, patients apply antibiotic ointment for 5 days to the donor area.

Hairline Design and Recipient Site Formation

As in every cosmetic procedure, realistic expectations need to be communicated to the patient during the initial consultation. The 2 most common goals of patients are a natural appearance and the achievement of maximum density, both of which are now described in terms of ethnic considerations.

The appearance of density is a factor of the following: the concentration of hairs (number of follicular units times the number of hairs in each follicular unit in a given area); the thickness or caliber of each hair; the color contrast between the hair and the scalp; and the angulation of the hair with the scalp (the more acute the angle, the greater the appearance of density). Some of the characteristics that maximize density also help with providing a more natural appearance (less color contrast between scalp and hair, more acute angulation), whereas others are associated with making appearances more difficult (thick caliber hairs) (**Fig. 2**). Probably in no ethnic group is this shown so well as in the Asian patient, in whom the color contrast between the hair and the scalp and the geometry of the hair make the achievement of density and natural appearances more difficult (**Fig. 3**). The opposite holds for the African American patient, in whom the curl of the hair and the similarities in color between the scalp and the hair make the achievement of density easier

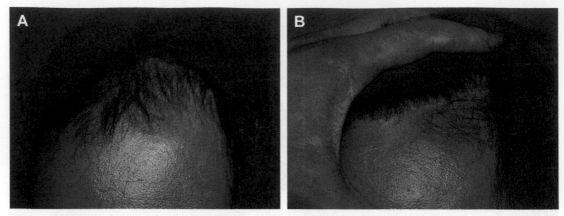

Fig. 2. Before (*A*) and 1 year after (*B*) FUG/strip procedure on Hispanic man. Note the irregular hairline with hairs acutely angled anterior.

(**Fig. 4**). With the East Indian and dark-skinned Hispanic and Middle Eastern individual, the lack of color contrast helps with density and naturalness (**Figs. 5–7**).

The recipient sites in patients of African and Asian ethnicity tend to be larger than those for average hair of whites. This difference is caused by the geometry and the thickness of the hair follicles. Whether obtained by FUE or FUG, follicles are preserved in their naturally occurring follicular units, and recipient sites are sized so that they match up with the size of the grafts. For fine-haired patients, 0.5-mm blades work for single-hair grafts, 0.6 and 0.7 mm for 2-hair grafts, and 0.7 and 0.8 mm for 3-hair grafts, In Asians and most East Indians, each of these blades needs to be 0.1 to 0.2 mm larger. In most African patients, these recipient sites also tend to need to be larger. Asian hairline design is treated similarly to the white hairline, in that sites are made in an irregular-regular manner to mimic a natural hairline.

In the African American patient, although the single-hair grafts tend to fit into 0.6-mm recipient sites, 2-hair grafts and 3-hair grafts are typically planted into recipient sites 0.8 to 1 mm in size, primarily because the grafts are large as a result of the curliness of the hairs. This curl of the African hairs allows for a hairline to appear natural.

Although beyond the scope of this article, natural appearing hairlines are generally created by the irregular distribution of single-hair grafts into small irregularly made triangles. Behind these several rows of single-hair grafts, 2-hair then 3-hair and 4-hair grafts are successively placed. An exception to this irregular triangle distribution is typically in patients of African ethnicity, in whom a more even, straighter hairline is usually preferable, because the curliness of the hairs makes the hairline appear natural. In Asian patients, it is rare to use grafts larger than 2 hairs, because of the unnaturalness that can be created by the use of 3-hair grafts, except in the most unusual

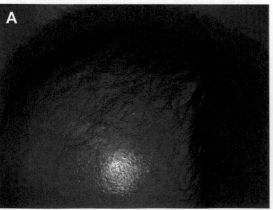
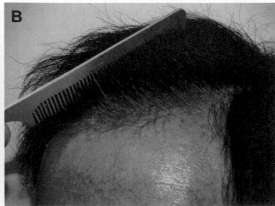

Fig. 3. Before (*A*) and 18 months after (*B*) FUG/strip procedure on Asian man. To achieve naturalness, most of the grafts consisted of 1-hair and 2-hair follicular units.

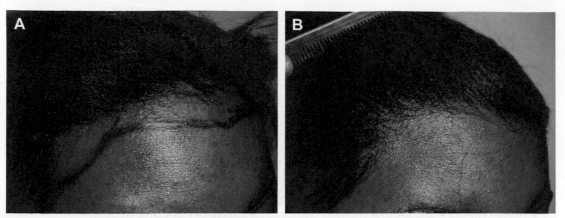

Fig. 4. Before (*A*) and 1 year after (*B*) FUG/strip procedure on African woman for hairline lowering.

circumstances. For the same reason, in no other ethnic group is forward angulation of grafts more imperative. Likewise, in African patients, this forward angulation is not so important because of the curl of the hairs.

Planting grafts into the recipient sites can be more challenging in patients of East Asian ethnicity, because of the challenges in visualizing the sites. For reasons that are unknown, the grafts of Pakistani patients tend to be soft or mushy, making them more difficult to plant. This difficulty is exacerbated because these patients tend to

have a higher incidence of bleeding from the recipient sites.

HAIR GRAFTING TO THE BEARD

This procedure has increased dramatically in popularity over recent years. This popularity increase has 3 causes: the popularity of American men sporting beards (epitomized by the Brooklyn hipster trend, which goes beyond white urban America); the information provided through the Internet as well as a deluge of media coverage

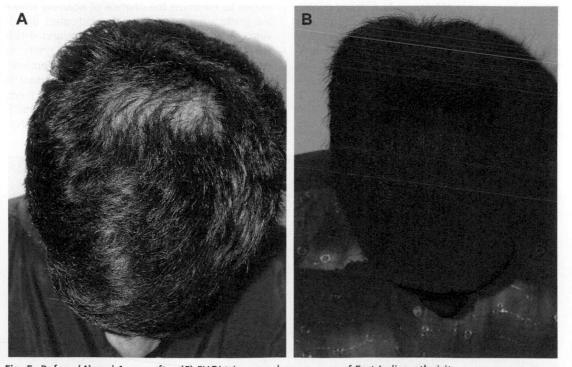

Fig. 5. Before (*A*) and 1 year after (*B*) FUG/strip procedure on man of East Indian ethnicity.

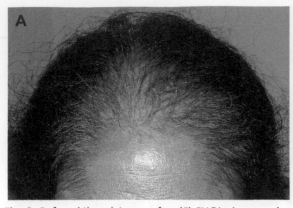 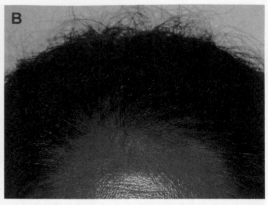

Fig. 6. Before (A) and 1 year after (B) FUG/strip procedure on woman of East Indian ethnicity.

that this procedure is available; and the not insignificant numbers of men of certain ethnicities desiring fuller beards. In addition, consistent with the increasing numbers of men in general seeking hair transplantation procedures because of the availability of the FUE technique, part of the growth in requests for beard transplantation is from men who shave or cut the scalp hair very short who also want more facial hair.

Hair transplantation to the beard consists of transplanting hair from usually the scalp to the face, where the hairs continue to grow (just like regular facial hair); if the procedure is performed properly and aesthetically, the hairs appear natural. A wide variety of requested patterns is desired, ranging from longer sideburns, to a strong goatee and mustache, to a narrow strap beard, to a full thick beard, including sideburns and goatee/mustache. The most common cause of a deficiency of facial hair is genetics, but other less common reasons include scarring from trauma (eg, burns) or previous surgery (eg, cleft lip repair, skin cancer, facelifts) and previous laser hair removal.

Both the FUG and FUE techniques can be used for obtaining the donor hairs; FUE is becoming more popular. Similar to the ethnic considerations for choice of technique with scalp hair transplant procedures, men of African and Asian ethnicity are usually best served by the FUE technique (African American because of the popularity of shaving the hair short, Asians because the typically spiky direction of hair growth in the back of the head makes it more likely that even a well-healed narrow linear donor site scar could be visible at nearly any hair length).

Whether obtained by the FUE or FUG technique, preparation of the grafts for transplanting includes trimming the surrounding epithelium from the edges to minimize the chance of scarring where the grafts are placed, and when indicated, subdividing the naturally occurring 3-hair and 4-hair follicular units into 2-hair and 1-hair grafts to ensure a more natural nontransplanted appearance. This subdividing is especially important in patients who have thick straight donor hairs, such as Asian men, in whom every hair is particularly visible, given the combination of thick hair

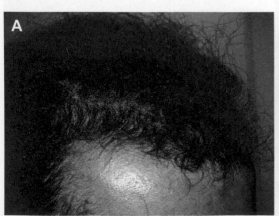 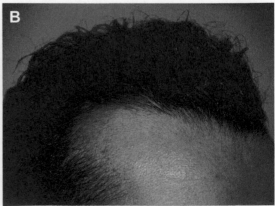

Fig. 7. Before (A) and 1 year after (B) FUG/strip procedure on man of Middle Eastern ethnicity.

caliber and the contrast of the dark hair color with light skin color, which is exacerbated because the goal of most Asian men is not a full thick beard but rather a well-defined but thin goatee or sideburns or strap beard, which leaves each graft to be more visible (**Fig. 8**). The transplanting of 3-hair (never 4-hair) naturally occurring FUGs can be beneficial to maximizing density in men with fine light-colored hairs or in some Middle Eastern and most East Indian men, in whom the goal is often the thickest possible beard (thus limiting the visibility of an individual graft), and many men of African ethnicity, in whom the curliness of the hairs makes them even less visible as individual follicular units.

Patients need to be aware that because the total number of donor hairs is limited, any hairs transplanted to the beard are no longer available for transplanting into the scalp into areas of existing or future male pattern baldness. The number of grafts needed for the face is a factor

of the areas to be filled in and the desired fullness and size of these areas (ie, narrow strap beard vs full cheek beard), which must be reconciled (and explained to the patient) with the safe number of available donor supply, keeping in mind the likelihood of further hair loss. The following is an approximate graft count needed for filling in areas of the face, and the number can be 40% higher or lower; higher, for example, when maximum coverage is desired (ie, Middle Eastern or East Indian men) or when donor hairs are thin in caliber (ie, more white or European Hispanic men); lower, for example, when only a thin amount of coverage is the goal (ie, Asian men):

Sideburns: 250 to 350 grafts per side
Mustache: 250 to 450 grafts
Full goatee (including mustache): 450 to 750 grafts
Cheek beard: 300 to 650 grafts per side

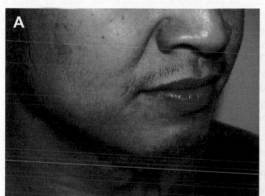

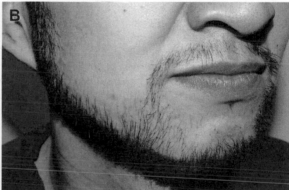

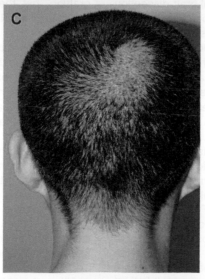

Fig. 8. Before (*A*) and 1 year after (*B*) FUE procedure to the beard on Asian man. Note the donor site at 1 year (*C*) free of detectable scarring.

One of the most important keys to achieving a natural appearing result is angling the recipient sites so that the transplanted hairs grow as flat as possible to the facial skin to avoid them sticking out from the face. This goal is best achieved by the use of the smallest possible recipient site blades (0.6 or 0.7 mm when possible; sometimes, 0.8 mm, when 3-hair grafts are used), which minimizes the rotational movement of the grafts with healing, thus keeping them at the intended angulation. It is imperative to keep the blade handle at this shallow angle to the facial skin, especially in the mustache, where the lip border often slightly protrudes because of the normal shape of the lip, which can undesirably push up on the blade handle.

Beard design varies tremendously amongst ethnic groups, because of ethnic considerations of masculinity as well as individual desires. For East Indian and Middle Eastern men, a thick beard is desired to enhance masculinity; for many men in India, this can improve the prospects of an arranged marriage; for some Hispanic men, a thick mustache is particularly desirable; for the Hassidic Jew, a beard is almost essential for social acceptance; for some Asian men, a well-defined yet not particularly dense sideburn as well as goatee, which can extend to a narrow strap beard that runs along the lower jawline, can provide a desired look, which is sported by some magazine models and actors.

HAIR GRAFTING TO THE EYEBROWS AND EYELASHES

Like with beard transplantation, restoring hair to the eyebrows depends on careful graft dissection and then placement in the proper angulation to achieve natural appearing results. Most eyebrow transplants are performed for women who have overplucked, but there are also men and women who have lost their eyebrows because of genetics, thyroid disease, trauma, and other causes.

The procedure typically requires the transplanting of primarily 1-hair, sometimes 2-hair grafts into recipient sites, made most commonly with a 0.5-mm width blade. These grafts are most often obtained by the FUG/strip technique, in which an incision 6 cm long can provide under microscopic dissection 600 to 750 grafts to allow for satisfactory filling in of the eyebrows. For patients who wish to keep their hair cut short, in particular African American men, and those at risk for a visible donor site scar, such as Asian men with coarse hair that is spiky such that it grows more outward than downward from the scalp, it is best to obtain the grafts by the FUE technique. Caution

needs to be paid when dissecting down 2-hair and especially 3-hair FUGs to obtain the more typically desired 1-hair and occasionally 2-hair grafts, so that the surrounding supportive tissue is left intact to ensure hair regrowth.

As with other hair transplants, those individuals with dark straight hair with light-colored scalps are more challenging, because the color contrast enhances the visibility of each graft and also increases underlying skin show, which is associated with the appearance of lower density. Thick straight hair is also more challenging than hair that is fine or curly, because it is difficult to make straight hair lie flat and thus grow in a more anatomic direction. Given these criteria, it can be deduced that the patients who typically achieve the most aesthetic results are those of light complexion and light-colored hair, or hair that is fine, or those with dark curly hair, especially those of dark complexion, such as those of African ethnicity. Although the hairs are more difficult to harvest and dissect, and the grafts require more care in placement into recipient sites to ensure that the native curl complements the desired direction of hair growth flat onto the brow skin, these patients can expect good results (**Figs. 9** and **10**). Other ethnic groups in whom results are typically more impressive include East Indians and some Middle Eastern individuals of darker complexion, whereas working with many Asian patients can be the greatest challenge (**Fig. 11**).

HAIRLINE LOWERING SURGERY

There are 2 techniques for advancing the overly high hairline in women. The more common is hair grafting, but the SHA technique has a definite role, with several advantages. Also called the hairline lowering or forehead shortening procedure, SHA involves making an incision along the hairline, then advancing the entire frontal scalp by as much as 3 to 5 cm, excising the overlapped forehead skin so that the hairline is now in a lower position. Endotine hooks are inserted into the frontal bone, positioned so that they engage the galea to secure the frontal scalp into its forwardly advanced position, and then, the incision is reapproximated in a trichophytic fashion so that the hairs can grow through what is typically a fine line scar. Although the procedure is most often performed under local anesthesia and oral sedation, the occasional patient chooses twilight sedation. If desired, a browlift can be added, performed in the subfrontalis muscle plane, to achieve a more youthful appearance.

Although wide undermining is performed in the subgaleal plane back to the vertex and 2 or

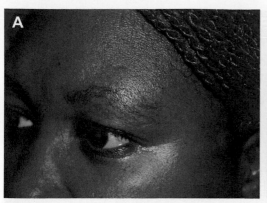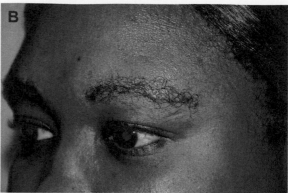

Fig. 9. Before (A) and 10 months after (B) eyebrow transplant on African woman.

3 galeotomies are made in the coronal plane to maximize the total amount of advancement, this procedure is indicated for patients with a flexible scalp that allows for sufficient advancement. Scalp laxity can be assessed by placing a finger on the midaspect of the prospective patient's hairline and observing how far anteriorly and posteriorly it can be moved, which approximates the amount of advancement that can be achieved, with each galeotomy typically adding another 2

to 3 mm. For patients with an inflexible scalp, if highly motivated, a cycle of balloon tissue expansion of the frontal scalp over a 4-week to 6-week period can allow for as much as 5 to 6 cm of additional advancement.

Other indications for SHA, in addition to a sufficiently mobile scalp, include a stable (nonthinning), reasonably dense frontal hairline, best assessed through physical examination and history. Patients with an inelastic scalp or thinning

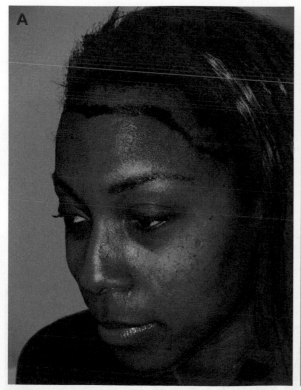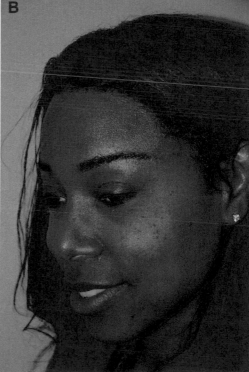

Fig. 10. Before (A) and 18 months after (B) FUG/strip procedure to advance hairline, along with eyebrow transplant, on African woman.

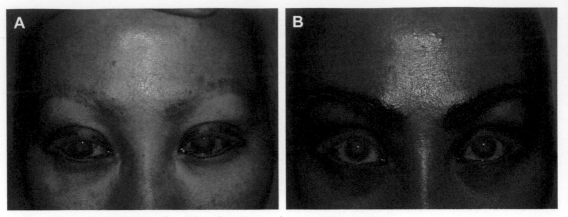

Fig. 11. Before (*A*) and 1 year after (*B*) eyebrow transplant on Asian woman.

hairline are better candidates for hair grafting. In addition, for patients who desire a more rounded hairline, hair grafting has to be performed, whether as a staged second procedure several months after SHA or as a stand-alone treatment. These hair grafts can also be transplanted into the hairline to both soften it as well as help further conceal the fine line scar that may be visible in the occasional patient.

SHA is appropriate for patients of all ethnicities but seems to be particularly popular for patients of African ethnicity. The reasons for this situation include the observed higher prevalence of genetically large foreheads associated with high hairlines that would require many grafts to sufficiently lower the hairline to where desired, and many African ethnicity patients having a mobile scalp that allows for 3 to 5 cm of advancement (**Fig. 12**).

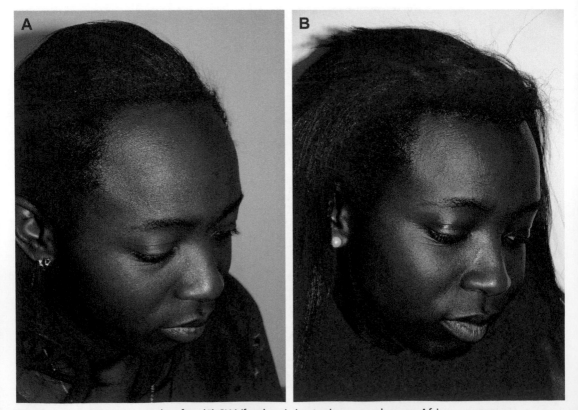

Fig. 12. Before (*A*) and 4 weeks after (*B*) SHA/forehead shortening procedure on African woman.

Hypertrophic or keloid scarring of the hairline incision does not seem to be a problem, and hair grafting can help conceal these fine line scars. Hair grafting in patients with dark skin (which blends in well with the dark hairs), whether of Hispanic, East Indian, or African ethnicity, usually results in a fuller look, a phenomenon enhanced with curly hair, making hair transplantation a good option to SHA. Similarly, light-colored hair coupled with fair skin color is another favorable combination for achieving denser appearances from hair grafting.

The more commonly chosen procedure to advance the overly high hairline is hair grafting. This is a typically less surgical procedure, involving the transplanting of 1200 to 2400 grafts (depending on how much lowering is desired) in a single procedure, taking 3 to 8 hours to perform (it is a meticulous procedure). Every graft is placed into tiny recipient sites (0.5–0.8 mm in size), each one made by the surgeon; these sites then determine the direction, pattern, and angulation of growth to ensure a natural appearance. The transplanted hairs typically fall out within 3 weeks, then start to regrow at 4 months, taking a full 10 months or longer for final results. The hair grafting procedure is ideal for hairlines that are thin or thinning out, for those who want a hairline that is not only lower but also more rounded, and for those who opt not to have or are not good candidates for SHA. Some patients desire a touch-up after 10 months or so to achieve greater density, but most do not need this touch-up.

REFERENCES

1. Franbourg A, Hallegot P, Baltenneck F, et al. Current research on ethnic hair. J Am Acad Dermatol 2003; 48(6):S115–9.
2. Richards GM, Oresajo CO, Halder RM. Structure and function of ethnic skin and hair. Dermatol Clin 2003;21:595–600.
3. Headington JT. Transverse microscopic anatomy of the human scalp: a basis for a morphometric approach to disorders of the hair follicle. Arch Dermatol 1984;120:449–56.
4. Sperling LC. Hair density in African Americans. Arch Dermatol 1999;135:656–8.
5. Kim JC. Asian hair: A Korean study. In: Pathomvanich D, Imigawa K, editors. Hair Restoration Surgery in Asians. Tokyo: Springer; 2010. p. 21–2.

Laser Skin Treatment in Non-Caucasian Patients

Amy Li Richter, MD[a], Jose Barrera, MD[b], Ramsey F. Markus, MD[c], Anthony Brissett, MD[d],*

KEYWORDS

- Laser • Skin • Resurfacing • Ethnic • Fitzpatrick • Hispanic • African American • Asian

KEY POINTS

- Ethnic skin presents a unique challenge for laser skin rejuvenation because of higher density of larger melanosomes, thicker collagen bundles, and increased fibroblast responses.
- Lasers may be safely used in patients with dark skin tones by choosing fractional technologies with longer wavelengths, lower fluences, and longer pulse durations.
- The risks of laser therapy include scarring, postinflammatory hyperpigmentation, and hypopigmentation.
- Developing careful treatment plans based on patient goals and maintaining careful attention to pre-procedural and postprocedural management strategies can minimize the risk of complications.
- In the hands of an experienced laser surgeon, laser resurfacing in dark skin types may improve the appearance of fine wrinkles and even skin tone, texture, and pigmentation.

INTRODUCTION

In the last decade, there has been an increase in the use of lasers for facial skin rejuvenation. Owing to improved technologies, patients are able to confront dermatologic concerns in an office-based setting with outpatient procedures. Conditions such as photoaging, acne vulgaris, and dyschromia can be treated with laser therapy, with improved risk profiles and decreased recovery times. Although the demand for facial rejuvenation and cosmetic procedures continues to increase among all ethnic populations and skin types, not all patients and skin types are the same and there is no one-size-fits-all treatment algorithm. In addition, the complications of therapy vary between skin types, and careful attention must be paid to these reaction patterns and specific treatment options.

Skin types and colors are divided into 6 photo-types, Fitzpatrick skin types I through VI, with I being the fairest and VI being the darkest (**Table 1**).[1] Within a single ethnicity, there may be variable phototypes, and it is important to tailor the treatment to the patient. The number of melanocytes is consistent throughout all ethnicities. Melanocytes derive from neural crest cells and transfer melanosomes, which contain melanin, into keratinocytes. The color of skin depends on the density, size, and activity of melanosomes, as darker skin has a higher density of larger melanosomes.[2] In addition, darker skin types, Fitzpatrick types V and VI, have thicker and more compact skin layers with thicker collagen bundles, which increase the epidermal barrier and reduce skin sensitivity (**Fig. 1**).[3,4] This barrier delays skin damage from the environment and ultraviolet

---

Disclosure: The authors A.L. Richter, MD, J. Barrera, MD, and A. Brissett, MD, have no significant financial or other relationships with commercial companies whose products may be discussed in this article. R.F. Markus, MD, discloses equipment loans from Lumenis LTD and Syneron-Candela Corporation.
[a] Bobby R. Alford Department of Otolaryngology–Head and Neck Surgery, Baylor College of Medicine, One Baylor Plaza NA 102, Houston, TX 77030, USA; [b] Department of Otolaryngology, San Antonio Military Medical Center, San Antonio, TX 78234, USA; [c] Department of Dermatology, Baylor College of Medicine, 1977 Butler Boulevard, Houston, TX 77030, USA; [d] Bobby R. Alford Department of Otolaryngology–Head and Neck Surgery, Baylor Facial Plastic Surgery Center, Baylor College of Medicine, One Baylor Plaza NA 102, Houston, TX 77030, USA
* Corresponding author.
E-mail address: brissett@bcm.edu

Facial Plast Surg Clin N Am 22 (2014) 439–446
http://dx.doi.org/10.1016/j.fsc.2014.04.006
1064-7406/14/$ – see front matter © 2014 Elsevier Inc. All rights reserved.

Table 1
Anatomy of skin types

Fitzpatrick Skin Type	Skin Characteristics	Sun Exposure
I	Pale white skin; blonde or red hair; blue eyes; freckles	Burns easily, never tans
II	White fair skin; blonde or red hair; blue, green, hazel eyes	Burns easily, tans minimally with difficulty
III	Cream white skin; any hair or eye color	Burns moderately, tans moderately and uniformly
IV	Moderate brown skin, Mediterranean	Burns minimally, tans moderately and easily
V	Dark brown skin, Middle Eastern	Rarely burns, tans profusely
VI	Deeply pigmented dark brown to black	Never burns, tans profusely

Adapted from Fitzpatrick TB. The validity and practicality of sun-reactive skin types I through VI. Arch Dermatol 1988;124:870.

radiation and aging in darker phototypes when compared with lighter skin types. Due to these histologic differences, dark skin is at increased risk for injury due to incidental laser absorption by melanin, problems with postinflammatory hyperpigmentation, and decrease in melanin production leading to hypopigmentation.

Although there are many types of lasers, the fundamental principle is the same: all lasers treat the skin by targeting a specific chromophore. The main chromophores of the skin are hemoglobin, melanin, and water. In general, resurfacing lasers are designed at specific wavelengths that use water as a chromophore to cause targeted thermal damage in the dermis to promote new collagen formation and skin tightening.[5] Other targetable chromophores include melanin, which has a broad, but

gradually decreasing, absorption coefficient from 250 to 1200 nm. The selection of a laser with a longer wavelength can allow for targeting of deep melanin or tattoo pigmentation in darker skin types.[4]

Other variables important to lasers include the thermal relaxation time, pulse duration, and energy fluence (**Table 2**). The thermal relaxation time is the time required for a tissue to cool to half temperature to which it was heated. Heating the tissue for time longer than the thermal relaxation time can cause thermal damage to surrounding tissue. In dark-skinned individuals, it is important to select a pulse duration longer than the thermal relaxation time of the epidermis but shorter than the target chromophore to avoid epidermal blistering, crusting, pigmentation changes, and scarring.[4] The fluence is the joules per square

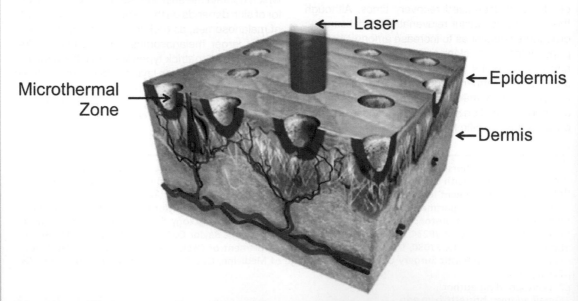

Fig. 1. Layers of the skin. The skin is divided into the epidermis, dermis, and hypodermis. Dark-skinned individuals have increased numbers of larger melanocytes, more compact skin layers, and thicker collagen bundles.

Table 2
Variables of lasers

Variable	Function	Example
Chromophore	Laser target molecule, unique absorption spectrum and peak absorption wavelength	Hemoglobin, melanin, water
Wavelength	Property of light measured in nanometers that influences how chromophores are targeted	Hemoglobin (variable absorption from 300 nm to infrared) Melanin (gradually decreasing absorption from 250 to 1200 nm) Water (1000 to 1 mm)
Thermal relaxation time	Time required for tissue to cool to half the temperature to which it was heated	Melanosome (250 ns) Vessels (2–10 ms) Hair follicles (100 ms)
Pulse duration	Time to heat tissue to target tissue; choose pulse duration less than or equal to thermal relaxation time of target chromophore to avoid damage to surrounding tissue	Pulse duration 10 to 100 ns to target melanosome
Energy fluence	Joules per square centimeter of energy emitted by a pulsed laser device	25 J/cm^2 used by a 1064-nm Nd:YAG for laser hair removal; highest tolerated fluences are 100 J/cm^2 (skin types IV, V) and 50 J/cm^2 (skin type VI)

centimeter of energy emitted from the laser handpiece. The laser fluence may need to be decreased to protect the epidermis to safely treat patients with darker skin types compared with those with lighter skin types. Other helpful strategies in safely treating patient of color include longer wavelengths, longer pulse durations, and skin cooling before, during, and/or after the procedure to avoid overheating the epidermis.[4,6]

CLASSES OF LASERS

The major classes of lasers include ablative and nonablative lasers in both nonfractionated and fractionated varieties (**Table 3**). Ablative lasers target water molecules in the epidermis, causing vaporization of skin cells and retraction of the dermis with collagen formation. Ablative lasers are more aggressive and function similar to a skin peel with prolonged recovery time and higher adverse event profile.[7] Nonablative lasers preserve the epidermis and target the dermal tissues to promote collagen formation. These nonablative treatments are milder and reduce the adverse event profile and recovery time. Fractionated lasers are designed to target microscopic treatment zones, or microthermal zones (MTZs) to create columns of thermal injury with adjacent normal skin.[4] This procedure promotes healing and improves skin texture compared with nonfractionated lasers without the high side-effect profile of ablative lasers. Radiofrequency resurfacing is a nonablative technique that uses a

low temperature to penetrate dermal tissues and promote collagen healing.[7] There are several options for laser therapy, and it is important to determine the expectations of your patient while balancing the risks and benefits associated with laser therapy in patient-specific phototypes.

TREATMENT GOALS

Lasers may be considered for a variety of indications, and the goals of the treatment should reflect the patient presentation.

Skin Laxity

There is an increased desire in all patients to achieve more youthful and refreshed facial skin. Over time, facial skin experiences photodamage, which causes wrinkles, texture changes, and abnormal pigmentation. Additional changes over time include soft-tissue volume loss, rhytides, and increased vascularity. The primary environmental factor that affects aging is ultraviolet radiation, but given the protective effects of melanin and a thicker epidermis, individuals with dark skin may experience less skin laxity due to gravity and volume loss compared with others with fair skin.[4]

Dyschromia

The primary concerns of patients may vary depending on ethnicity and skin type (**Fig. 2**). Dyschromia is a common presentation of dark-skinned patients, and it is important to

Table 3
Classes of lasers and clinical outcomes

Laser	Outcomes	Risks
Ablative nonfractionated • 10,600-nm CO_2 laser • 2940-nm Er:YAG laser • Combined CO_2 Er:YAG laser	Dramatic improvement in wrinkle reduction, alleviate acne and atrophic scars[7]	Oozing, bleeding, and crusting (100%)[7]; acne, transient hyperpigmentation and hypopigmentation (IV) (55%–68%)[7,8]; scarring and poor wound healing, permanent skin hypopigmentation[4,7]
Nonablative nonfractionated • 1319-nm pulsed dye laser • 1320-nm Nd:YAG laser • 1540-nm diode laser	Improvement scar severity (29%)[3]; improvement acne scars (10%–50%)[2,9]; atrophic scarring and acne-induced PIH (III–VI) (51%–75%)[5]; limited wrinkle improvement[2]	Minimal, few hours of erythema, no scaling or peeling, no abnormal pigmentation[7]
Nonablative fractionated • 1410-nm laser • 1440-nm Nd:YAG laser • 1540-nm laser • 1550-nm Er laser • 1927-nm thulium fiber laser	Moderate improvement in texture and wrinkles[4]; significant improvement in acne scarring (51%–75%)[3,5] and overall appearance: excellent (30%), significant (59%), moderate (11%)[3,9]; safe in dark skin types because of limited tissue damage and melanocyte stimulation[7]	Moderate downtime; moderate pain[5]; postinflammatory hyperpigmentation (III, IV, V) (3%, 12%, 33%, respectively)[5]; acne (2%)[8,10]; herpetiform eruptions (2%)[8,10]
Ablative fractionated • 10,600-nm fractional CO_2 laser • 2940-nm fractional Er:YAG laser • 1790-nm fractional Er:YSGG laser	Moderate resurfacing power for mild skin laxity and rhytides[2]; moderate improvement in photodamage, scars (37%), and dyspigmentation[2,7]	Moderate downtime, moderate complications[8]; postinflammatory hyperpigmentation (II–V) (44%)[3]; use with caution in skin type VI[2]

Abbreviation: PIH, post-inflammatory hyperpigmentation.
Data from Refs.[2–5,7–10]

distinguish between melasma and postinflammatory hyperpigmentation when considering laser therapy.[4,7,11–13] Options for laser treatment of dyschromia include the Nd:YAG laser and fractional nonablative devices.[7]

Laser Hair Removal

The use of lasers for hair removal relies on melanin absorption within the hair follicle (**Fig. 3**). Laser hair removal may be complicated in patients with dark skin because of unintended epidermal overheating leading to blistering, crusting, and subsequent pigmentary changes.[4] With this in mind, longer-wavelength lasers (1064-nm Nd:YAG) with lower fluences and skin cooling may be used successfully in darker skin types for the treatment of hypertrichosis.[2]

Keloids and Hypertrophic Scarring

Keloids and hypertrophic scars occur more commonly in dark-skinned individuals. Laser treatment of thickened scars may be considered in

combination with intralesional steroid injections.[4] The pulsed dye laser has been shown to decrease erythema, improve pain and pruritus, decrease lesion height, and improve hypertrophic scar pliability. These effects may facilitate intralesional steroid injection. However, the pulsed dye laser can target epidermal pigmentation and must be used with caution in patients with dark skin. Keloids may also be treated with the 1064-nm Nd:YAG laser with moderate results of mild keloids. The lesion is injected with intralesional triamcinolone 10 mg/mL up to 3 mL before starting therapy with regular laser treatments (fluence 13–18 J/cm^2, 2000 pulses) for 6 weeks.[2] After 7 weeks, the lesion may be reevaluated and treatment repeated if necessary.

PREPROCEDURAL PLANNING: MEDICAL OPTIMIZATION

Before embarking on laser rejuvenation of facial skin, it is important to emphasize routine skin

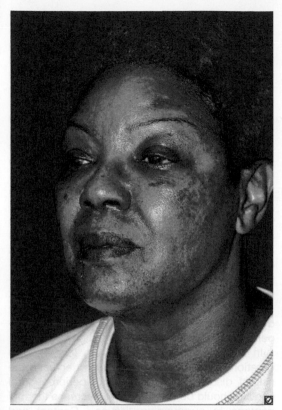

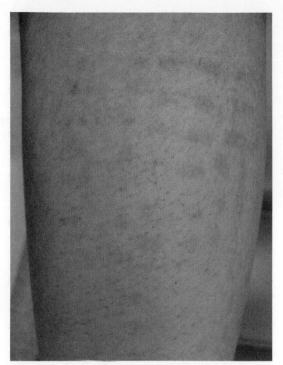

Fig. 3. Laser hair removal. Lasers can be used for treatment of hypertrichosis in all skin types by targeting the melanin chromophore in the hair follicle with a low risk of dyspigmentation.

Fig. 2. Dyschromia may present as hyperpigmentation or hypopigmentation and is one of the most common treatment goals of laser therapy in ethnic populations.

care to patients to optimize facial skin health before procedures. Sun should be avoided when possible, and mechanical and chemical blockade (broad-spectrum A and B sunscreens) should be used daily. Acne vulgaris can be treated with topical and oral antibiotics, hormonal treatments, and isotretinoin safely in all skin types and should be optimized before starting laser rejuvenation therapy.[8] However, all isotretinoin should be avoided for 6 to 12 months before starting laser therapy due to the possibility of poor healing. In addition, all herpes simplex virus (HSV) outbreaks should be treated with antivirals, and prophylaxis antivirals should be given to patients with HSV before starting laser treatments.

Additional topical treatments with melanin suppressors, such as hydroquinones, kojic acid, azeleic acid, or emblica, may be considered for treatment of dyspigmentation and melasma before laser treatments, particularly in dark phototypes where nonablative laser therapies require a series of treatments to achieve satisfactory results.[4]

When considering laser treatment on a patient with dark skin, a test spot adjacent to the intended area of treatment may be performed, as individuals of the same ethnicity and phototype may react differently to the laser depending on variable skin characteristics.[14] Test spots should be started at low-density, low-fluence, and longer-pulse-duration settings. Full response and side effects should be observed at 1 month, at which point scarring and pigment changes will likely be evident.

PROCEDURAL APPROACH: CHOOSING A LASER

For historical reasons, one should note the ablative nonfractionated lasers, including the 10,600-nm carbon dioxide (CO_2) laser, the 2940-nm erbium-doped yttrium aluminum garnet (Er:YAG) laser, and the combined CO_2 Er:YAG laser (see **Table 3**). These lasers target the water molecules in the dermis and vaporize the epidermis. This laser has the most significant outcomes with significant improvement of fine wrinkles and acne scars.[9] However, side effects are a significant issue with this category of devices and include acne, permanent hypopigmentation, temporary hyperpigmentation, skin infections, and scarring. For these reasons, ablative nonfractionated lasers should be used with extreme caution in patients with

Fitzpatrick type IV skin and are contraindicated in phototypes V and VI because of the increased risk of dyspigmentation and scarring (occasionally keloidal).[4]

Due to the side-effect profile of the ablative nonfractionated lasers, a more gentle approach using nonablative technology was developed. The nonablative nonfractionated lasers include the 1319-nm pulsed energy laser, the 1320-nm neodyminum-doped YAG laser (Nd:YAG), and the 1450-nm diode laser. These lasers have had slight improvement with skin resurfacing and good results with acne treatment.[1] There is minimal recovery required with these lasers, little erythema, and minimal peeling. The nonablative nonfractionated lasers often require serial treatment sessions (4–6 treatments) to obtain improvement but can be used safely in patients with dark skin because of decreased risk of scarring and dyspigmentation.[7]

To more effectively treat the skin, nonablative fractionated lasers were developed to combine a more aggressive pulse and the safety of fractionation while still avoiding the epidermal loss incurred with ablative lasers. These include the 1410-nm laser, the 1440-nm Nd:YAG laser, the 1540-nm laser, the 1550-nm erbium laser, and the 1927-nm thulium fiber laser. These nonablative fractionated lasers frequently require several treatments (2–6), with moderate improvements in skin tone and texture with moderate downtime.[7] The targeting of tiny diameter and deep dermal penetration of each MTZ allows for stimulation of collagen formation while avoiding disruption of the epidermal barrier function.[9] These lasers can be used safely in dark phototypes with a small risk of temporary hyperpigmentation.

The ablative fractionated lasers are the most recent addition to the laser family. These lasers were developed in an attempt to increase resurfacing effectiveness while still enjoying quicker healing with fewer complications compared with ablative nonfractionated resurfacing. These include the 10,600-nm fractional CO_2 laser, the 2940-nm fractional Er:YAG laser, and the 2790-nm fractional erbium-doped yttrium scandium gallium garnet (Er:YSGG) laser. These lasers target MTZs with ablation and vaporization of dermal and epidermal tissues. A series of sessions may give resurfacing results nearly comparable to the ablative nonfractionated lasers but with much improved safety profiles.[7] These lasers can improve skin laxity and mild rhytides, but due to the violation of the epidermal layer, there is a risk of infection, scarring, and dyspigmentation and should be used with caution in patients with Fitzpatrick type IV through VI skin.[7]

Radiofrequency technologies achieve mildly improved facial skin tone and texture by denaturing existing dermal collagen and stimulating new collagen through low temperatures and deep tissue penetration. This option decreases the risk of dyspigmentation and scarring, and patient discomfort is minimal.[2,7]

When choosing a laser for hair removal, the 1024-nm Nd:YAG is the safest choice in dark-skinned individuals because the wavelength is poorly absorbed by melanin, which reduces the damage to dark epidermal pigmentation.[2] In addition, the pulse length can be adjusted to deliver the pulse over a longer period to facilitate cooling. Other laser choices for hair removal include the alexandrite and diode lasers at lower fluences and wider pulse widths. As with laser treatment of other skin disorders, multiple treatment sessions may be needed to achieve permanent results. Risks of laser hair removal in Fitzpatrick skin types IV to VI include blistering and temporary dyspigmentation, with a low risk of permanent hyperpigmentation or hypopigmentation.[2,3]

In addition to using lasers with longer pulse duration and longer wavelength to decrease the risk of discoloration or scarring, periprocedural cooling should be considered to decrease thermal damage to surrounding tissues.[3] Contact and noncontact cooling have the added benefit of improving patient comfort during laser therapy while decreasing thermal damage to the epidermis without interfering with laser intensity and direction. Options for contact cooling include skin moistening, application of ice or ice packs, and laser-specific cooling tips.[6]

POSTPROCEDURAL CARE AND FOLLOW-UP

The importance of postprocedural planning and skin care cannot be overstated when managing patients after laser treatment. Because many of these treatments often require several sessions, reducing skin damage between treatments can optimize epidermal healing and dermal collagen regeneration. The skin is more sensitive than usual for a short time after laser treatment, and sun blockade and cooling agents should be used judiciously. Darker phototypes have more reactive and labile fibroblasts compared with skin types I to III, and further dermal injury should be avoided.[2]

After laser treatment and depending on the type of laser used, mild erythema, edema, peeling, and flaking may occur and typically resolve over several days.[10] The period for full recovery depends on the exact type of laser treatment, and postoperative care must be tailored to the treatment administered. The postoperative skin care routine should include keeping the skin clean and moist to allow for reepithelization and to minimize the potential of scarring. In general, chilled saline-soaked gauze is applied intermittently for the first several days. The treated area should be gently treated with a mild cleanser such as Cetaphil, followed by the application of an oxygen-permeable ointment such as Aquaphor. Patients should be encouraged not to pull or pick at their skin as it starts to flake or peel, as this may increase the likelihood of scarring. Depending on the type of laser or resurfacing technique used, reepithelization typically occurs within a week. Avoidance of sun and the liberal use of sunscreen should be encouraged. Patients should avoid the use of retinoids and other bleaching agents for risk of causing irritation.

Most laser patients feel a sunburnlike sensation for the rest of the day after laser therapy. Topical skin care, oral analgesics, and cooling agents can all be used to improve patient comfort. Topical cooling agents, such as ice packs, are encouraged postprocedurally to improve patient comfort and decrease inflammation. Topical steroids may be considered in patients with persistent erythema.

POTENTIAL COMPLICATIONS AND MANAGEMENT

Careful patient selection combined with conservative and judicious implementation of laser treatments can result in positive outcomes when dealing with patient of color and dark skin types. In this particular subset of patients, the most common postprocedural concerns are related to dyspigmentation and scarring.

Postinflammatory hyperpigmentation is a common occurrence with ablative laser options and is a bothersome side effect in darker phototypes (Fitzpatrick skin types V–VI) (**Fig. 4**).[2,7] There are several options for topical therapies when considering the treatment of hyperpigmentation, such as hydroquinone, azeleic acid, kojic acid, and emblica. Hydroquinone, a common treatment option, is a plant-derived tyrosinase inhibitor and is often used to treat discrete hyperpigmented patches.[4] Deleterious outcomes related to the use of hydroquinone may include hypopigmentation surrounding the treated area because of adjacent bleaching, in a halo effect.[2,10]

Delayed hypopigmentation is a less common complication usually seen after ablative nonfractionated laser resurfacing several months after treatment (**Fig. 5**). This complication is permanent and a major cause for avoiding ablative nonfractionated resurfacing in dark-skinned patients. This condition can be confused with hypopigmentation

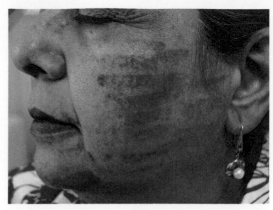

Fig. 4. Posttreatment postinflammatory hyperpigmentation. Postinflammatory hyperpigmentation is common with ablative lasers and may be reduced by using nonablative and fractionated techniques.

attributed to the use of retinoids and hydroquinone before laser treatment, which resolves with discontinuation of the medication.[10]

In addition to dispigmentation after laser treatment, additional complications such as acneiform eruptions and HSV infections may occur in all skin types (**Fig. 6**).[8] Acne eruptions are more common in patients with acne-prone skin and can be minimized by premedicating with oral antibiotics such as tetracycline. In general, prophylactic antivirals are recommended in patients with a history of orofacial HSV. When treating patients with a history of HSV outbreaks with laser exposure, antivirals should be started before the initiation of laser therapy and continued up to a week after laser application. Laser rejuvenation should not be performed on patients with active HSV infections.

Although bacterial superinfections are uncommon, they should be treated aggressively to minimize scarring and dyspigmentation.[8,10] Bacterial

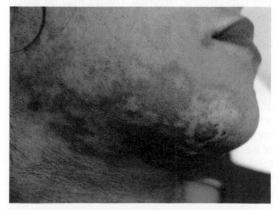

Fig. 5. Posttreatment hypopigmentation. Hypopigmentation after laser therapy is a rare complication that may present several months after treatment.

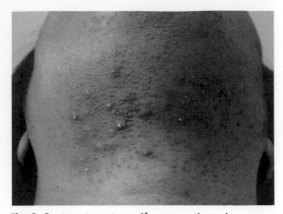

Fig. 6. Posttreatment acneiform eruptions. A common complication after laser therapy is acneiform eruptions and HSV infections. This risk can be minimized with premedication in select patients with skin types predisposed to such infections.

superinfections typically present with pain, increased erythema, exudates, erosions, and crusting. Infections should be cultured and treated with broad-spectrum oral antibiotics to reduce long-term risk of scarring. When treating patients of dark skin types, the development of acne eruptions, HSV infection, or bacterial superinfections can intensify the likelihood of pigment issues and discoloring of the soft-tissue envelope. Every effort should be made to prevent these complications or treat them aggressively should they occur.

SUMMARY

Ethnic skin presents a unique challenge for laser skin rejuvenation because of higher density of larger melanosomes, thicker collagen bundles, and increased fibroblast responses. Special considerations need to be made when considering laser therapy for ethnic patients for the treatment of skin laxity, dyschromia, hypertrichosis, keloids, and hypertrophic scarring. Lasers may be safely used in patients with dark skin tones by choosing fractional technologies with appropriate wavelengths, lower fluences, longer pulse durations, and maintaining careful attention to preprocedural and postprocedural management strategies. When considering the use of lasers, the treatment goals should reflect individual patient complaints and the realistic expectations of laser skin rejuvenation. Patients should be counseled on the risks of laser therapy, including scarring, postinflammatory hyperpigmentation, and hypopigmentation. With this in mind and in the hands of an experienced laser surgeon, laser resurfacing in darker

skin types IV through VI may eliminate unwanted hair, improve the appearance of fine wrinkles, and even skin tone, texture, and pigmentation.

REFERENCES

1. Fitzpatrick TB. The validity and practicality of sun-reacitve skin types I through VI. Arch Dermatol 1988;124:869–71.
2. Woolery-Lloyd H, Viera MH, Valins W. Laser therapy in black skin. Facial Plast Surg Clin North Am 2011; 29:405–16.
3. Alexis AF. Lasers and light-based therapies in ethnic skin: treatment options and recommendations for Fitzpatrick skin types V and VI. Br J Dermatol 2013;169(Suppl 3):91–7.
4. Rossi AM, Perez MI. Laser therapy in Latino skin. Facial Plast Surg Clin North Am 2011;19:389–403.
5. Carniol PJ, Woolery-Lloyd H, Zhao AS, et al. Laser treatment for ethnic skin. Facial Plast Surg Clin North Am 2010;18:105–10.
6. Tierney EP, Hanke CW. The effect of cold-air anesthesia during fractionated carbon-dioxide laser treatment: prospective study and review of the literature. J Am Acad Dermatol 2012;67:436–45.
7. Preissig J, Hamilton K, Markus R. Current laser resurfacing technologies: a review that delves beneath the surface. Semin Plast Surg 2012;26: 109–16.
8. Graber EM, Tanzi EL, Alster TS. Side effects and complications of fractional laser photothermolysis: experience with 961 treatments. Dermatol Surg 2008;34:301–5.
9. Doherty SD, Doherty CB, Markus JK, et al. A paradigm for facial skin rejuvenation. Facial Plast Surg 2009;25:245–51.
10. Metelitsa AI, Alster TS. Fractionate laser skin resurfacing treatment complications: a review. Dermatol Surg 2010;35:299–306.
11. Davis SA, Narahari S, Feldman SR, et al. Top dermatologic conditions in patients of color: an analysis of nationally representative data. J Drugs Dermatol 2012;11:466–73.
12. Ho SG, Chan HH. The Asian dermatologic patient: review of common pigmentary disorders and cutaneous diseases. Am J Clin Dermatol 2009; 10:153–68.
13. Davis EC, Callender VD. Postinflammatory hyperpigmentation: a review of the epidemiology, clinical features and treatment options in skin of color. J Clin Aesthet Dermatol 2010;3:20–31.
14. Cole P, Hatef D, Kaufman Y, et al. Laser therapy in ethnic populations. Semin Plast Surg 2009;23: 173–7.

Laser and Face Peel Procedures in Non-Caucasians

Mark J. Been, MD[a,b], Devinder S. Mangat, MD[a,b,c,*]

KEYWORDS

- Ethnic skin • Non-ablative lasers • Superficial peels • Facial resurfacing

KEY POINTS

- Non-Caucasian skin types represent a significant percentage of patients who seek facial resurfacing procedures.
- Inherent within non-Caucasian skin types is the increased risk for complications from lasers and chemical peels, including dyspigmentation and scarring.
- Traditional ablative lasers have largely been replaced by nonablative and fractional lasers.
- Chemical peels for non-Caucasian skin types are typically limited to superficial depths.
- Common reasons non-Caucasian patients seek resurfacing are dyschromias, including melasma and postinflammatory hyperpigmentation, acne scarring, facial rejuvenation, keloids and hypertrophic scars, cutaneous lesions, and hair-related conditions.

INTRODUCTION

More than ever there is growing popularity in facial resurfacing and rejuvenation, as the goal to maintain one's youthful and attractive features becomes increasingly important. Historically, facial resurfacing procedures were described in the treatment of fair-skinned individuals of European descent, corresponding to Fitzpatrick skin types I to III (**Table 1**).[1] With the advent of new technologies and resurfacing techniques, there is increased potential to treat those of darker, non-Caucasian skin types. A 2013 national survey by the American Society of Aesthetic Plastic Surgery revealed that 22% of surgical and nonsurgical aesthetic procedures were performed on non-Caucasians (Hispanics, 8%; African Americans, 7%; Asians, 6%; other, 1%).[2] For the purposes of this discussion, non-Caucasian skin will be considered Fitzpatrick skin types IV to VI. This population poses unique circumstances and

challenges that must be recognized by the provider to achieve successful outcomes. Within this article we discuss various laser and light modalities, as well as chemical peels, used for facial resurfacing in non-Caucasian skin types.

Multiple definitions of beauty exist across cultures worldwide; however, several variables are universal: uniform distribution of skin pigment; smooth, tight skin; and an absence of rhytids are cornerstones of a youthful appearance and are the premises that facial resurfacing is based on.

Facial skin aging occurs via intrinsic and extrinsic pathways. Intrinsic changes are due to an individual's genetics, immune and general medical status, and include volume loss from lipoatrophy, gravitational sagging of skin, and resorption of the bony facial skeleton. Extrinsic changes include skin color aberrations, pigment redistribution in the form of lentigines, rhytids, actinic damage, elastic skin changes, and keratoses.[3] Smoking, exercise, and nutritional status

Disclosures: The authors have no financial or other considerations to disclose.
a Private Practice, 133 Barnwood Drive, Cincinnati, OH 41017, USA; b Private Practice, 56 Edwards Village Boulevard, Edwards, CO 81632, USA; c Department of Otolaryngology Head and Neck Surgery, University of Cincinnati, 222 Piedmont Avenue, Cincinnati, OH 45219, USA
* Corresponding author. 133 Barnwood Drive, Edgewood, KY 41017.
E-mail address: devindermangat5@gmail.com

Facial Plast Surg Clin N Am 22 (2014) 447–452
http://dx.doi.org/10.1016/j.fsc.2014.04.012

Table 1
Fitzpatrick skin type classification

Classification	Skin Color	Tanning Pattern	Burning Pattern
Type I	Very white	Never tans	Always burns
Type II	White	Tans minimally	Usually burns
Type III	White to olive	Tans moderately	Sometimes burns
Type IV	Light brown	Tans readily	Rarely burns
Type V	Dark brown	Tans profusely	Very rarely burns
Type VI	Black	Tans profusely	Never burns

contribute to extrinsic changes; however, the most important factor in extrinsic skin aging is ultraviolet (UV) photodamage.[4]

In setting the goals of treatment, one must take into consideration the unique histologic differences between Caucasian and non-Caucasian skin types. Although the absolute number of melanocytes is similar across races, darker skin pigment is the result of increased amounts of melanin within the skin. Within lighter skin types, the melanin is located in melanosomes within melanocytes confined principally to the stratum basale layer of the epidermis. In non-Caucasian skin, there are increased numbers of melanosomes with increased levels of melanin. The melanosomes also are more widely distributed throughout the epidermis.[5] Cadaveric studies of black-colored skin biopsies have demonstrated an average sun protective factor of 13.4.[6] Other findings in darker skin types include relatively thicker skin and increased fibroblast activity.[7] Findings such as these support the clinical observations that photoaging, particularly rhytids, in darker skin types tends to lag 1 to 2 decades behind that of the fair skin counterparts.

LASER AND LIGHT MODALITIES

The historic standard resurfacing laser therapies relied on ablative CO_2 and erbium-doped yttrium aluminum garnet (Er:YAG) lasers. These modalities are usually reserved for fair-skinned individuals (Fitzpatrick skin types I–III). As mentioned previously, there are a number of histologic findings unique to non-Caucasian skin. These findings also are responsible, in part, for causing increased

risk of complications, namely dyspigmentation and scarring. Melanin is a chromophore with a wide light absorption spectrum (250–1200 nm). Absorption tends to be greater at shorter wavelengths and less at longer wavelengths. Because there is a greater amount of melanin distributed throughout the epidermis, increased laser energy absorption results in greater heat production and subsequent thermal tissue injury.[7]

For these reasons, darker-skinned individuals are treated primarily with newer laser and light technologies, including nonablative, fractional, and wide-spectrum light modalities. Nonablative lasers selectively target the dermis while the epidermis is spared, aided by direct skin cooling. Additionally, lower fluences and longer pulse durations help to minimize thermal injury and subsequent complications.[8] Commonly used nonablative lasers include neodymium (Nd):YAG (1064 nm), 1450-nm diode, and pulsed dye laser (PDL) (585–595 nm). Nonablative erbium-doped fractional laser (1550 nm) and ablative fractional CO_2 (10,600 nm) lasers rely on creating microthermal zones (MTZ) surrounded by untreated tissue, thereby reducing overall tissue injury and allowing rapid recovery time. When fractional therapies are used, fractional treatment densities can be lowered to minimize risk. Intense pulsed light (IPL) (515–1200 nm) uses a broad range of wavelengths and can treat a variety of conditions in non-Caucasian skin. The trade-off when using the more conservative modalities to minimize complications is that less overall tissue destruction occurs and resultant tissue regeneration and remodeling are less significant than that attained in more aggressive treatments of fair-skinned individuals. As a result, more treatment sessions are often required.

CHEMICAL PEELS

As with laser and light therapies, to perform chemical peels on non-Caucasian individuals, one must recognize the trade-off between achieving the desired clinical improvements and minimizing the risk of postinflammatory hyperpigmentation (PIH), hypopigmentation, and scarring. For this reason, the general practice is limited to superficial chemical peels for patients with Fitzpatrick skin types IV to VI. Superficial peels are defined as those that induce tissue destruction limited to the epidermis with inflammation reaching as deep as the superficial papillary dermis. Healing is expected within 3 to 5 days, and the usual side-effect profile is limited to mild peeling, erythema, and mild burning pain. Medium and deep peels carry too great a risk of postoperative complications; therefore, they are almost always withheld from non-Caucasian patients. Commonly used superficial peels include alpha-hydroxy acids, namely glycolic acid (10%–70%), as well as salicylic acid (20%–30%), trichloroacetic (TCA) acid (10%–30%), and Jessner solution.[9] It should be noted that the frost typically marking the end point in TCA peels for fair-skinned patients should be avoided in dark-skinned patients, as this may confer increased risk of dyspigmentation and scarring.

PATIENT SELECTION AND PREPARATION

As with any patient encounter, the initial consultation provides an opportunity to thoroughly assess the patient's history and physical examination. One must address patient concerns, establish realistic expectations, and, ultimately, decide on the appropriateness to pursue the resurfacing procedure. For non-Caucasian patients, in particular African American patients, a personal and family history of keloid and hypertrophic scar formation should caution the practitioner from aggressive resurfacing. Because of the increased risk of dyspigmentation and scar formation, any use of exogenous hormones, recent use of isotretinoin or photosensitizing drugs, or an active inflammatory state (eg, herpes simplex labialis) should be considered contraindications. PIH can be particularly pronounced in ethnic skin types; therefore, patients must be counseled about the need for postoperative sunlight avoidance and strict adherence to preoperative and postoperative care regimens.

Up to 6 weeks before resurfacing, patients can be started on topical therapies to increase the rate of epithelialization, stabilize melanocyte activity, and reduce local inflammation. Typically a combination composed of topical retinoids, such as tretinoin, hydroquinone, and topical steroids is used. The authors use a topical preparation of 0.025% tretinoin, 8% hydroquinone, and 1% hydrocortisone. In treatment of pigmentation, meta-analysis has demonstrated superior improvement with triple combination therapy (tretinoin, hydroquinone, topical steroid) than with monotherapy alone.[10] Topical therapy is stopped 3 to 4 days before the procedure, but may be restarted 1 week after the procedure. Oral antiherpetic prophylaxis is initiated 3 days before resurfacing and continued 5 to 7 days until reepithelialization is complete.

For both laser and chemical peel resurfacing, test spots should be performed to assess the patient's response to the intended therapy. Laser test spots should begin with the most conservative settings and gradually progress to the desired

strength. Test spots should be performed on skin similar to the area to be resurfaced.

COMMONLY TREATED CONDITIONS
Dyschromias

Melasma and PIH are the most common dyspigmentations in dark-skinned individuals and represent one of the most common reasons non-Caucasians seek treatment. Melasma is an acquired dyschromia resulting in hyperpigmented areas of skin. The etiology is thought to result from increased size rather than number of melanocytes.[11] The cause is unknown; however, this condition is observed to more readily affect non-Caucasian skin types.[12] Melasma can be exacerbated by excessive UV radiation, exogenous hormone intake, pregnancy, and photosensitizing drugs. PIH is another focal alteration in skin pigmentation, the result of increased deposits of melanin in the epidermis and/or dermis following an inflammatory process. This may be the result of postprocedural inflammation or can be secondary to various inflammatory or hypersensitivity-mediated skin processes.

Initial treatment for dyschromias involves topical depigmenting therapies, often with antityrosinase activity, such as hydroquinone. Prompt initiation of treatment, as well as UV protection, is paramount to prevent worsening of PIH. Chemical peels may be initiated when topical therapy is ineffective. Ten percent to 70% of glycolic acid peels and 20% to 30% of salicylic acid peels are effective in treating both melasma and PIH.[13–16] Ten percent to 30% of TCA peels and Jessner solution have demonstrated efficacy in treatment of melasma, although their effects in treatment of PIH are not well documented.[17–19]

Laser resurfacing is another treatment option for refractory cases of melasma and PIH. Manaloto and Alster[20] studied the effects of the ablative Er:YAG laser. Fluences of 5.1 to 7.6 J/cm^2 were used to successfully treat melasma. PIH almost always occurred at 3 to 6 weeks after treatment, but successfully resolved with glycolic acid peels. Nonablative fractional photothermolysis and IPL have both been used to treat melasma in non-Caucasians.[21] The fractional laser is approved by the Food and Drug Administration for treatment of melasma.[16] Recommendations for treatment using nonablative Er-doped fractional laser include an energy level of 15 mJ and density of 125 MTZ cm^{-2} per pass with a total of 8 passes.[22,23] Q-switched pigment-specific lasers have been used to treat PIH. The Q-switched Nd:YAG laser has been found effective in treatment of PIH in East Asian populations (Fitzpatrick skin types IV and V).[24] IPL and fractional lasers offer promising new modalities to treat PIH; however, there is concern for persistent hyperpigmentation and further studies are warranted.

Acne Scars and Photoaging

Non-Caucasian skin types are prone to significant sequelae of persistent acne, such as scarring and dyspigmentation.[25] Diffuse facial acne scars are traditionally treated with CO_2 and Er:YAG ablative lasers, as well as deep chemical peels, although this practice is seldom used for darker skin types. Instead, nonablative and fractional lasers have increased in prevalence. Nd:YAG (1320 nm), 1450-nm diode, and Er:glass (1540 nm) are frequently used, as these longer-wavelength lasers penetrate to the dermis and avoid epidermal melanin absorption.[8] The 1450-nm diode laser has been found effective in treating atrophic facial scars in Asians with Fitzpatrick skin types IV and V.[26]

The nonablative Er-doped fractional laser is used for acne scarring. Recommended ranges for energy and treatment densities for non-Caucasian skin types are 40 to 70 mJ and 200 to 392 MTZ cm^{-2}.[27] A head-to-head retrospective review from Saudi Arabia compared acne scar improvement between the nonablative 1550-nm Er-doped fractional laser and the ablative fractional CO_2 laser in non-Caucasian skin types. At least 50% improvement in the acne scars was attained in 35% of the nonablative group and 37% of the ablative group. Incidence of PIH was 17% in the nonablative group and 14% in those using the ablative CO_2 laser.[28]

Although the effects of photodamage are often less pronounced and occur later in life in non-Caucasian skin types, signs of photodamage, namely facial rhytids and mottled pigmentation, become more apparent. The aforementioned nonablative and fractional lasers and superficial chemical peels may be used for these indications. IPL has also demonstrated efficacy in East Asian populations.[3] Because of the superficial nature of these treatment modalities, deeper rhytids present difficult challenges. A primary concern remains the development of PIH, which may occur in up to 40% of nonablative, 33% of fractional nonablative, and 92% of fractional ablative laser cases.[29,30] Combination peels, such as TCA with glycolic acid, may improve acne scars and mottled pigmentation but pose an increased risk because of deeper dermal penetration.[31]

Keloid and Hypertrophic Scars

Although ablative CO_2 and Er:YAG lasers may be used to treat recalcitrant keloids and hypertrophic

scars, the risk of unsightly dyspigmentation and recurrence may be unacceptably high.[8] PDL is an effective nonablative means to target oxyhemoglobin and theoretically disrupt blood flow within scar tissue to inhibit fibroblast activity. Conell and Harland[32] studied the effect of PDL followed by intralesional steroid injection and found an overall 60% improvement in lesion height, 40% improvement in erythema, and 75% improvement in pain and itching. A recent meta-analysis of 28 clinical trials compared the efficacy of various lasers in treatment of keloid and hypertrophic scars.[33] The 532-nm laser systems and the 585/595-nm PDL laser demonstrated the best response rates, although the PDL results were better in fair-skinned individuals. These findings may further signify the importance of oxyhemoglobin absorption and photothermolysis in treatment of keloids and hypertrophic scars.

Cutaneous Lesions

Cutaneous masses in darker skin can be successfully reduced or flattened with resurfacing procedures. Syringomas, dermatosis papulosa nigra, and vascular lesions are observed in darker skin types. Syringomas have been successfully reduced with TCA peels and ablative CO_2 lasers.[34] Dermatosis papulosa nigra, notably found in the periorbital region and histologically similar to seborrheic keratoses, has been improved with the 1064-nm Nd:YAG, potassium titanyl phosphate, and nonablative 1550-nm fractional lasers.[35] Vascular lesions, such as telangiectasias and hemangiomas, may be managed with nonablative lasers, such as PDL or Nd:YAG, to minimize epidermal melanin absorption; however, success rates are mixed.[36]

Hair-Related Conditions

Hypertrichosis, and other hair-related disorders common to darker-skinned individuals, including pseudofolliculitis barbae and acne keloidalis nuchae, may be addressed with laser and peel modalities. Hair removal in darker skin requires the laser to target the melanin within the hair bulb but avoid absorption from melanin in the surrounding epidermis. Long pulse durations, lower fluences, longer-wavelength lasers, and diligent epidermal cooling allow the hair follicle to be selectively destroyed.[37,38] The 800-nm to 810-nm diode, intense pulsed light, and long-pulsed 1064-nm Nd:YAG lasers are commonly used for hypertrichosis in darker-skinned individuals.[22,39,40] A prospective, randomized trial between the long-pulsed Nd:YAG laser and intense pulsed light showed significant reduction in hair counts at 6 months with both modalities. Side-effect profiles were similar; however, the long-pulsed Nd:YAG laser was deemed more effective by both the patients and evaluator.[41]

Pseudofolliculitis barbae is more common in individuals with curly hair in regions where the hair is shaved or plucked. African American individuals are particularly prone to PIH resulting from this condition. Salicylic and glycolic acid peels are effective in treatment of pseudofolliculitis barbae.[31,42] A series of multiple treatments is typically necessary to achieve clinical improvement. Serial treatments using a low-fluence (12 J/cm^2) setting with the 1064-nm Nd:YAG laser has demonstrated significant reduction in dyspigmentation, papules, and textural changes.[43] Acne keloidalis nuchae, also known as folliculitis keloidalis nuchae, predominantly affects the occipital scalp and posterior neck of Afro-Caribbean male individuals. Long-standing lesions predispose this group to hypertrophic scars and keloids. Treatment is largely medical; however, the 1064-nm Nd:YAG laser may be used to treat this condition.

SUMMARY

Despite the increased risk of complications observed in non-Caucasian skin types, laser resurfacing and chemical peels remain viable treatment options for a number of skin conditions. The practitioner should understand the need for more conservative treatment in this group of patients. When unexpected sequelae, such as PIH occur, prompt treatment with diligent follow-up will expedite resolution. Pretreatment and posttreatment with melanocyte-stabilizing and anti-inflammatory agents, as well as UV avoidance and protection are advised.

REFERENCES

1. Fitzpatrick TB. The validity and practicality of sun-reactive skin types I-VI. Arch Dermatol 1988;124:869–71.
2. The American Society for Aesthetic Plastic Surgery. Cosmetic Surgery National Data Bank Statistics. 2013. Available at: http://www.surgery.org/sites/default/files/Stats2013_3.pdf. Accessed April 22, 2014.
3. Davis EC, Callender VD. Aesthetic dermatology for aging ethnic skin. Dermatol Surg 2011;37(7):901–17.
4. Brissett AE, Naylor MC. The aging African-American face. Facial Plast Surg 2010;26(2):154–63.
5. Taylor SC. Skin of color: biology, structure, function, and implications for dermatologic disease. J Am Acad Dermatol 2002;46(Suppl 2):S41–62.
6. Kaidbey KH, Agin PP, Sayre RM, et al. Photoprotection by melanin—a comparison of black and Caucasian skin. J Am Acad Dermatol 1979;1:249–60.
7. Herd RM, Dover JS, Arndt KA. Basic laser principles. Dermatol Clin 1997;15:355–72.
8. Cole PD, Hatef DA, Kaufman Y, et al. Laser therapy in ethnic populations. Semin Plast Surg 2009;23(3):173–7.
9. Salam A, Dadzie OE, Galadari H. Chemical peeling in ethnic skin: an update. Br J Dermatol 2013;169(Suppl 3):82–90.
10. Rivas S, Pandya AG. Treatment of melasma with topical agents, peels and lasers: an evidence-based review. Am J Clin Dermatol 2013;14(5):359–76.
11. Grimes PE, Yamada N, Bhawan J. Light microscopic, immunohistochemical and ultrastructural alterations in patients with melasma. Am J Dermatopathol 2005;27:96–101.
12. Davis EC, Callender VD. Postinflammatory hyperpigmentation: a review of the epidemiology, clinical features, and treatment options in skin of color. J Clin Aesthet Dermatol 2010;3(7):20–31.
13. Rendon M, Berneburg M, Arellano I, et al. Treatment of melasma. J Am Acad Dermatol 2006;54(Suppl 2):S272–81.
14. Burns RL, Prevost-Blank PL, Lawry MA, et al. Glycolic peels for postinflammatory hyperpigmentation in black patients: a comparative study. Dermatol Surg 1997;23:171–4 [discussion: 175].
15. Grimes PE. The safety and efficacy of salicylic acid chemical peels in darker racial ethnic groups. Dermatol Surg 1999;25:18–22.
16. Grimes PE. Management of hyperpigmentation in darker racial ethnic groups. Semin Cutan Med Surg 2009;28:77–85.
17. Nanda S, Grover C, Reddy BS. Efficacy of hydroquinone (2%) versus tretinoin (0.025%) as adjunct topical agents for chemical peeling in patients of melasma. Dermatol Surg 2004;30:385–9.
18. Ejaz A, Raza N, Iftikhar N, et al. Comparison of 30% salicylic acid with Jessner's solution for superficial chemical peeling in epidermal melasma. J Coll Physicians Surg Pak 2008;18(4):205–8.
19. Safoury OS, Zaki NM, El Nabarawy EA, et al. A study comparing chemical peeling using modified Jessner's solution and 15% trichloroacetic acid versus 15% trichloroacetic acid in the treatment of melasma. Indian J Dermatol 2009;54(1):41–5.
20. Manaloto RM, Alser T. Erbium:YAG laser resurfacing for refractory melasma. Dermatol Surg 1999;25:121–3.
21. Wang CC, Hui CY, Sue YM, et al. Intense pulsed light for the treatment of refractory melasma in Asian persons. Dermatol Surg 2004;30(9):1196–200.
22. Alexis AF. Lasers and light-based therapies in ethnic skin: treatment options and recommendations for Fitzpatrick skin types V and VI. Br J Dermatol 2013;169(Suppl 3):91–7.

23. Tierney EP, Hanke CW. Review of the literature: treatment of dyspigmentation with fractionated resurfacing. Dermatol Surg 2010;36:1499–508.

24. Kim S, Cho KH. Treatment of facial postinflammatory hyperpigmentation with facial acne in Asian patients using a Q-switched neodymium-doped yttrium aluminum garnet laser. Dermatol Surg 2010;36:1374–80.

25. Taylor SC, Cook-Bolden F, Rahman Z, et al. Acne vulgaris in skin of color. J Am Acad Dermatol 2002;46(Suppl 2):S98–106.

26. Chua SH, Ang P, Khoo LS, et al. Nonablative 1450-nm diode laser in the treatment of facial atrophic acne scars in type IV to V Asian skin: a prospective clinical study. Dermatol Surg 2004;30(10):1287–91.

27. Alexis AF. Fractional laser resurfacing of acne scarring in patients with Fitzpatrick skin types IV-VI. J Drugs Dermatol 2011;10(Suppl 12):S6–7.

28. Alajlan AM, Alsuwaidan SN. Acne scars in ethnic skin treated with both non-ablative fractional 1,550 nm and ablative fractional CO2 lasers: comparative retrospective analysis with recommended guidelines. Lasers Surg Med 2011;43(8):787–91.

29. Lee HS, Lee DH, Won CH, et al. Fractional rejuvenation using a novel bipolar radiofrequency system in Asian skin. Dermatol Surg 2011;37(11):1611–9.

30. Graber EM, Tanzi EL, Alster TS. Side effects and complications of fractional laser photothermolysis: experience with 961 treatments. Dermatol Surg 2008;34(3):301–5 [discussion: 305–7].

31. Roberts WE. Chemical peeling in ethnic/dark skin. Dermatol Ther 2004;17(2):196–205.

32. Conell PG, Harland CC. Treatment of keloid scars with pulsed dye laser and intralesional steroid. J Cutan Laser Ther 2000;2(3):147–50.

33. Jin R, Huang X, Li H, et al. Laser therapy for prevention and treatment of pathologic excessive scars. Plast Reconstr Surg 2013;132(6):1747–58.

34. Frazier CC, Camacho AP, Cockerell CJ. The treatment of eruptive syringomas in an African American patient with a combination of trichloroacetic acid and CO2 laser destruction. Dermatol Surg 2001;27:489–92.

35. Polder KD, Landau JM, Vergilis-Kalner IJ, et al. Laser eradication of pigmented lesions: a review. Dermatol Surg 2011;37(5):572–95.

36. Stratigos AJ, Alora MB, Uroste S, et al. Cutaneous laser surgery. Curr Probl Dermatol 1998;10:127–74.

37. Ross EV, Cooke LM, Timko AL, et al. Treatment of pseudofolliculitis barbae in skin types IV, V, and VI with a long-pulsed neodymium:yttrium aluminum garnet laser. J Am Acad Dermatol 2002;47(2):263–70.

38. Battle EF Jr. Advances in laser hair removal in skin of color. J Drugs Dermatol 2011;10:1235–9.

39. Vachiramon V, Brown T, McMichael AJ. Patient satisfaction and complications following laser hair removal in ethnic skin. J Drugs Dermatol 2012;11(2):191–5.

40. Breadon JY, Barnes CA. Comparison of adverse events of laser and light-assisted hair removal systems in skin types IV-VI. J Drugs Dermatol 2007;6:40–6.

41. Ismail SA. Long-pulsed Nd:YAG laser vs. intense pulsed light for hair removal in dark skin: a randomized controlled trial. Br J Dermatol 2012;166(2):317–21.

42. Perry PK, Cook-Bolden FE, Rahman Z, et al. Defining pseudofolliculitis barbae in 2001: a review of the literature and current trends. J Am Acad Dermatol 2002;46(Suppl 2):S113–9.

43. Schulze R, Meehan KJ, Lopez A, et al. Low-fluence 1,064-nm laser hair reduction for pseudofolliculitis barbae in skin types IV, V, and VI. Dermatol Surg 2009;35(1):98–107.

Scar Treatment Variations by Skin Type

Marty O. Visscher, PhD[a,b,*], J. Kevin Bailey, MD[c], David B. Hom, MD[d]

KEYWORDS

• Scar • Skin color • Melanin • Pigmentation • Hypertrophic • Keloid • Laser • Ethnicity

KEY POINTS

- Patients and clinicians use skin color attributes such as color uniformity, color distribution, and texture to infer physiologic health status.
- Normalization of skin color, surface texture, and height are important treatment goals.
- Skin color, structure, function response to trauma, and scar formation vary with ethnicity.
- The incidence of hypertrophic and keloid scar formation is influenced by these inherent variations.
- Skin type influences the response to various modalities including laser therapy and surgical intervention, and skin differences must be considered in treatment planning to achieve optimal results.

INTRODUCTION

Deep tissue wounds, burns, and surgical incisions can result in the formation of scars, that is, erythematous, firm, pruritic, raised fibrous masses that remain within the boundaries of the original wound, and may regress over time.[1] Scars frequently have significant morbidity and psychological, cosmetic, and functional outcomes as well as overall quality of life.[2] Patients seek treatment to improve the color, texture, surface roughness, pliability, range of motion functionality, and pain.

This paper discusses the impact of skin color and ethnicity on the physiologic characteristics of scars and on the evaluation of treatment efficacy. The implications of ethnic diversity in the selection of treatment strategies are examined.

SKIN COLOR

Clinical judgments of scar progression and treatment effectiveness depend on perception of the skin surface.[3] Humans use skin color attributes such as color uniformity, color distribution, and texture to infer physiologic health status.[4–8] In one study, subjects were asked to adjust the red color of high-resolution facial images to achieve a "healthy appearance". All of them increased the red color, regardless of the inherent pigmentation, but dark skin subjects increased the red color of dark skin photos more than lighter skin photos.[4] Visual responses to facial images standardized for shape and surface features were measured. Images with more uniform skin coloration were perceived to be younger than those with greater

Funding Sources: None.

Conflict of Interest: None.

[a] Skin Sciences Program, Division of Plastic Surgery, Cincinnati Children's Hospital Medical Center, 3333 Burnet Avenue, Cincinnati, OH 45229, USA; [b] Department of Surgery, College of Medicine, University of Cincinnati, Cincinnati, OH 45267, USA; [c] Division of Trauma, Critical Care and Burn, Wexner Medical Center, The Ohio State University, 410 West 10th Avenue, Columbus, OH 43210, USA; [d] Division of Facial Plastic & Reconstructive Surgery, Department of Otolaryngology-Head & Neck Surgery, University of Cincinnati College of Medicine, Cincinnati, OH 45267, USA

* Corresponding author. Skin Sciences Program, Division of Plastic Surgery, Cincinnati Children's Hospital Medical Center, 3333 Burnet Avenue, Cincinnati, OH 45229.

E-mail address: Marty.visscher@cchmc.org

facialplastic.theclinics.com

color variability.[9] These factors can reduce the perceived age by as many as 20 years.[10,11] The perception of age may vary however depending on the viewer's ethnicity. High-resolution images of facial skin (cheek region) of Japanese women aged 13 to 80 years were perceived to be older by Japanese observers if the skin was darker (L value) and more yellow (b*).[12]

Perceived skin color occurs when visible light interacts with skin components such as constitutive pigments melanin (yellow to brown), oxygenated hemoglobin (red), deoxyhemoglobin (blue-purple), bilirubin (yellow), and carotene (yellow).[13] Observed color arises from the interplay of light with components of the stratum corneum (SC), epidermis, and dermis and by diffuse reflection, scattering, and absorption of light inside the skin.[13,14] About 5% of incident light is reflected back to the eye, whereas the remainder is absorbed, scattered, or transmitted within the SC, epidermis, dermis, and subcutaneous tissue.[6] The SC transmits light, the epidermis and dermis absorb some light due to melanin and hemoglobin, and the subcutaneous fat scatters light.[15] The Vancouver Scar Scale (VSS), commonly used to evaluate scars, infers vascularity from color descriptors, pigmentation from color due to melanin, height relative to the surrounding tissue, and pliability by palpation.[16]

SKIN STRUCTURE, FUNCTION, COLOR, AND ETHNIC DIVERSITY

Skin color is commonly described by 2 systems:

1. Fitzpatrick skin type
2. Von Luschan skin coloration

The Fitzpatrick skin type system has 6 classifications based on inherent color and the response to ultraviolet radiation.[17] An anthropologist, Fredrick Von Luschan, described skin coloration in the late 1900s.[18] **Fig. 1**, and **Table 1** compare these systems in relation to skin color.

Melanin, water, hemoglobin, and other chromophores absorb the incident light to varying extents, depending on the wavelength. Melanin synthesis occurs in the basal layer of the epidermis and is transferred to the keratinocytes throughout the epidermis.[19] Melanin levels are higher in dark versus light skin and the latter has greater amounts of light melanin including pheomelanin and dihydroxyindole-2-carboxylic acid–enriched eumelanin.[20] Additionally, African skin is characterized by significantly larger melanosomes than Indian, Mexican, Chinese, and European skin and size is greater in Indian than in European skin.[20,21] Oxygenated blood in the dermal capillaries and vascular plexus and deoxygenated blood (blue-purple) in the dermal venules contribute to skin color.[22] Bilirubin (yellow) in the epidermis results from precipitation in phospholipid membranes and leakage as a complex with albumin into extravascular regions.[23] Skin coloration for a given individual varies with season due to differences in the amount of light exposure.[24]

Melanin (M) content can be approximated from measurements of red reflectance using the equation $M = \log_{10} (1/\% \text{ red reflectance})$, and erythema (E) can be determined from the equation $E = \log_{10} (1/\% \text{ green reflectance}) - \log_{10} (1/\% \text{ red reflectance})$.[25,26] Narrow band reflectance spectroscopy and CIE $L^*a^*b^*$ tristimulus color have been used to measure erythema, melanin, L^*, and a^* in various ethnic skin types (**Fig. 2**).[25] For subjects with lesser pigmentation, E and M are relatively independent and can be used to estimate erythema and melanin content. However, because E and M are correlated, they cannot be used to assess redness or melanin content for dark-skinned subjects.

Most of the published reports on ethnic skin comparisons have focused on the SC and epidermis rather than on exploring dermal and subcutaneous features.[27] The vascular response to a topical corticosteroid (clobetasol) using laser Doppler technique was decreased in African Americans versus Caucasians and paralleled the reduction in erythema in earlier studies by the same investigators.[28] The mechanism responsible for this effect was not discussed. Evaluations of three-dimensional reconstructed dermal equivalents and human tissue samples found the dermal-epidermal junction from African skin to have more epidermal projections, greater convolution, and to be more uniform than in Caucasian skin.[27] African tissues had lower amounts of laminin 5, nidogen proteins, type IV collagen, and type VII collagen than Caucasians. The syntheses of keratinocyte growth factor and monocyte chemotactic protein-I were higher in African papillary fibroblasts.

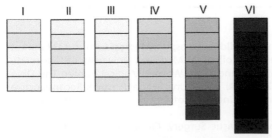

Fig. 1. The skin colors described by Von Luschan are shown in relationship to the Fitzpatrick skin types I to VI.

Table 1 Skin color classifications			
Fitzpatrick Type	Description	Effect of Light Exposure	Von Luschan's Schema[18]
I	Pale, fair, freckles	Always burns, never tans	Very light
II	Fair	Usually burns, sometimes tans	Light
III	Light brown	May burn, usually tans	Intermediate
IV	Olive brown	Rarely burns, always tans	Mediterranean
V	Brown	Moderate constitutional pigmentation	Dark or brown
VI	Black	Marked constitutional pigmentation	Very dark or black

Adapted from Weller R, Hunter J, Savin J, et al. Cinical dermatology. 4th edition. Malden (MA): Blackwell Publishing; 2008.

SCARS AND SKIN TYPE

Tissue injuries can result in significant inflammation including increases in cells eg, neutrophils, macrophages, monocytes, growth factors, and cytokines that stimulate fibroblast migration and proliferation, excessive collagen and extracellular matrix deposition culminating in the formation of a hypertrophic scar.[29] These scars have fine, well-organized type III collagen bundles, containing fibroblasts, numerous myofibroblasts, endothelial cells, and a higher density of microvesssels.[30–32] Examples of hypertrophic scars are provided in **Fig. 3.**

The incidence of hypertrophic scars from burn injury ranges from 32% to 78%, and the risk factors are dark skin, female gender, age (younger), time to heal, injury severity, neck or upper limb site, and a higher number of surgeries.[33] For pediatric patients undergoing reconstructive and release surgeries, scarring at the donor site can be more severe than in the original injury.[34] An evaluation of the effect of ethnicity on hypertrophic

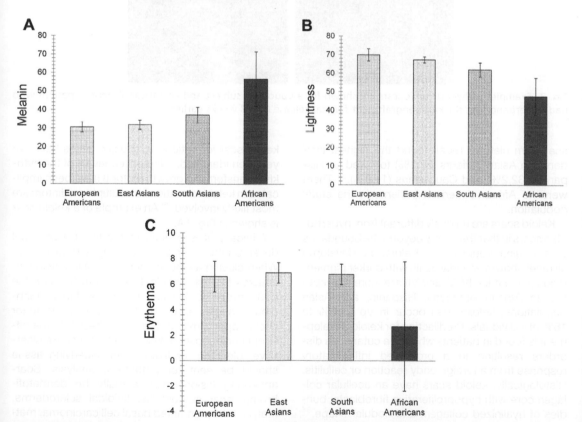

Fig. 2. Melanin content (*A*), skin lightness (*B*), and skin erythema (*C*) values measured from reflectance spectroscopy are shown for 4 ethnic groups: European Americans, East Asians, South Asians, and African Americans.

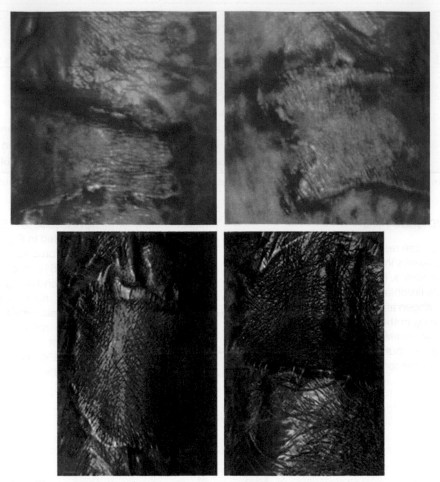

Fig. 3. Examples of hypertrophic scars are shown for a Caucasian subject and an African American patient who had undergone split thickness engraftment for scar release 6 to 8 weeks earlier.

scar from cleft lip repair found the highest incidence in Asian patients (36.3%) followed by Hispanics (32.2%) and Caucasians (11.8%).[35] There were no African American patients in the study population.

Keloid scars are uniquely different from hypertrophic scars in that they grow beyond the boundaries of the original wound area.[36] Keloids can develop in all races; however, individuals with darker pigmentation (Fitzpatrick IV, V, and VI) are more susceptible. In African American, Hispanic, and Asian populations, keloids can occur in up to 6% to 16% of individuals. Predilection for keloid development is found in patients who have cutaneous disorders resulting in a prolonged inflammatory response from a foreign body reaction or cellulitis. Histologically, keloid scars have an acellular collagen core with hypoproliferative fibroblasts, bundles of hyalinized collagen, and nodular shape.[36] Immune cells have also been identified in keloid tissue.[37] There is a strong genetic susceptibility for keloid scar formation but specific genes have not yet been identified.[38] Increased levels of the cytokine transforming growth factor β have been implicated in keloid formation but multiple mediators are most likely involved.[39] An example of a keloid scar is shown in **Fig. 4**A.

Clinically, it is difficult to predict if a scar will develop into either a keloid or hypertrophic scar. When closing a wound, increased skin tension increases the risk of keloid formation. Sites on the body prone to keloids are the earlobes, mandibular angle, upper back, shoulders, posterior neck, upper arms, and anterior chest.[40] In the differential diagnosis of keloids, scars that are ulcerative, bleeding, or fixed to its underlying tissue should be sent for pathologic analysis. Scar-appearing lesions may actually be dermatofibroma, scar sarcoidosis, keloidal scleroderma, morpheic or pigmented basal cell carcinoma, metastatic skin nodules, and dermatofibrosarcoma protuberans.

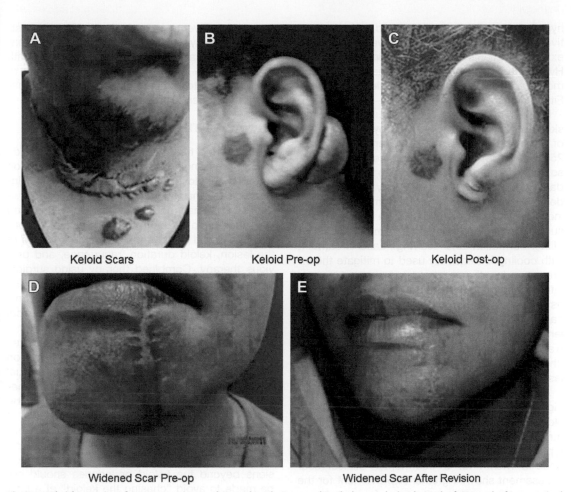

Fig. 4. Keloid scars in African American subjects (*A, B*). Frames (*B, C*) show a keloid scar before and after surgical treatment. Frames (*D, E*) show a widened scar on the chin before and after surgical correction.

SCAR MANAGEMENT

Optimization of coloration is an important goal of scar treatment.[41,42] Multiple modalities have been used for scar management, including glucocorticoid injections, retinoic acid, application of silicone gels, pressure garments, and simple massage.[43–48] Application of intense pulsed light (IPL), photothermolysis with pulsed dye laser (PDL), and ablation with a fractional CO_2 laser are used to normalize scar color, size, and pliability.[49,50] In randomized within-subject controlled study, one-half of newly healed skin grafts received PDL treatments at 6-week intervals in patients from a pediatric burn facility.[51] The entire scar was treated with compression per the standard of care. Decreases in quantitative scar erythema and height and an increase in tissue elasticity were observed after 2 or 3 treatments for the PDL plus compression treatment versus compression alone. VSS scores showed improvement for vascularity, pliability, pigmentation, and height

for PDL plus compression versus compression alone. Scars improved (VSS scores) following PDL treatment of linear operative scars 3 times beginning on the day of suture removal.[52]

Clayton and colleagues[49] reported on laser-based treatment of 95 patients with burn scars beginning 6 months post-injury. A combination of laser modalities was used to optimize outcome. In general, the initial treatment was with a 595-nm flashlamp-pumped PDL (7 mm spot, cryogenic cooling 30-msec spray, 20-msec delay, pulse duration 1.5 msec, overlapping 30%) beginning at fluencies of 5.0 to 8.0 J/cm². After mitigation of hyperemia, the protocol used a fractional CO_2 laser (density 15%, frequency 600 Hz, 12.5–17.5 mJ pulse) to decrease thickness and reduce stiffness. Superficial ablation (frequency 150 Hz, 70–90 mJ per micropulse) was applied to improve texture. An IPL laser (filter 515–590 nm, fluence 18–24 J/cm²) was used to normalize pigmentation and treat folliculitis. The incidence of hypopigmentation and hyperpigmentation was 12% and 2%, respectively. Adverse events were observed to a greater extent in patients with higher Fitzpatrick scores. Hypopigmentation and blister formation occurring more frequently compared with patients with lower Fitzpatrick scores.

Laser treatment of scars, particularly in darker-skinned patients, is confounded by the presence of melanin because it absorbs energy in region of 250 to 1200 nm (**Fig. 5**).[53] The pigment melanin absorbs some of the laser energy, up to 40% in very dark skin[54] and, therefore, may diminish the desired effect on the scar. Compensation by increasing the power increases the heat to the tissue and can result in thermal damage, including blister formation and scarring. Laser treatment with cooling is frequently used to mitigate the increases in tissue temperature but post-inflammatory hyperpigmentation has been noted as a side effect of cooling.[55] Melanin absorption can be reduced by using lasers with longer wavelengths where its absorption is lower. Longer wavelengths penetrate deeper into the dermis (the 810-nm diode laser and the 1064-nm Nd:Yag laser).

A within subject controlled trial compared 2 higher wavelength lasers, a long-pulsed 1320-nm Nd:Yag system and a 1450-nm diode laser, on atrophic facial scars among patients of Fitzpatrick types I to V.[56] One half was treated with each laser once a month for 3 treatments. Clinical scar assessment showed greater improvement for the 1450-nm laser, and quantitative surface roughness (measured by the 3D Primos system) decreased significantly for both lasers at 3, 6, and 12 months after treatment was complete. Both resulted in increased dermal collagen by histology at 6 months and this remained the same after 12 months. Twenty percent of patients had post-inflammatory hyperpigmentation. The use of nonablative fractional lasers at a lower density but with twice as many treatments decreased the risk of post-inflammatory hyperpigmentation in Asian patients who received treatment of acne scars.[57]

MANAGING THE ELUSIVE KELOID

Presently, the treatment management of keloids remains challenging and elusive. Surgical excision with primary closure, followed by local steroid injection is the mainstay of treatment (**Box 1**). However, the optimal treatment of keloids on the head and neck remains controversial. Factors to consider for keloid treatment are the site and size of the lesion, keloid duration, recurrence, and previous therapy. Combined therapy using surgical excision, post-operative steroid injection, and silicone sheeting has a 15% recurrence rate.[58] Examples of keloid scars before and after surgical intervention are shown in **Fig. 4**B–E.

In removing a keloid for the first time, the edges should be closed primarily with minimal tension on the surrounding skin. All sources of residual inflammation such as trapped hair follicles, epithelial cysts, and dermal sinus tracts should be removed to prevent recurrent keloid growth. If the keloid is large, serial excision should be considered to minimize excessive skin tension leaving a small perimeter of keloid behind. Making incisions beyond the keloid boundaries should not be made to avoid "chasing the keloid" at a later date. Corticosteroid injection can be given at the time of surgery and at monthly intervals for 4 to 6 months. The choice of using a scalpel versus a laser depends on the surgeon's personal preference. Local skin flaps, Z-plasties, and W-plasties

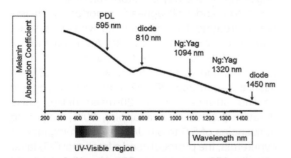

Fig. 5. The absorption coefficient of melanin at various wavelengths of energy. Laser treatment of scars, particularly in darker-skinned patients, is confounded by the presence of melanin because it absorbs energy in region of 250 to 1200 nm. The energies of various lasers used in the treatment of scars are indicated. (*Data from* Battle EF Jr, Soden CE Jr. The use of lasers in darker skin types. Semin Cutan Med Surg 2009;28(2):130–40.)

Box 1
Common primary treatments for keloid scars

Common Primary Treatments

  Surgical excision

  Laser (CO_2, 585 nm pulsed dye)

  Steroid injection

  Cryotherapy

Adjunctive Treatments

  Steroid injection

  Radiotherapy

  Mechanical pressure

  Silicone sheeting/gel

  Mitomycin C, 5-fluorouracil

should be avoided beyond the defect to prevent a larger keloid recurrence. Other methods of primary treatment are cryotherapy and the use of lasers (CO_2, 585 nm pulsed dye), which are described in following paragraphs regarding patients with Fitzpatrick IV, V, and VI.

Cryotherapy uses a refrigerant to flatten the keloid by inducing cell and microcirculatory damage leading to tissue necrosis and sloughing. Two to ten sessions separated by 25 days may be needed to diminish the keloid. Cryotherapy is often combined with intralesional steroid injection with an 84% keloid response. A side effect of cryotherapy is hypopigmentation due to cold sensitivity of melanocytes; this is especially relevant to darker-pigmented patients who are at increased risk for hypopigmentation. Furthermore, postprocedure healing can be prolonged requiring several weeks.[59]

When considering laser excision, increased melanin within the epidermis of a more darkly pigmented individual will interfere with the absorption of laser energy intended for another target, leading to hyperpigmentation of the treated area. History of isotretinoin use should be obtained as laser treatment could lead to atrophy of the sebaceous glands and potentially more scarring. In African American, Mediterranean, and Southeast Asian patients, histories of disorders such as sickle cell anemia, thalassemia, and glucose-6-phosphate dehydrogenase deficiencies should be obtained because these hereditary hemolytic diseases may affect post-operative healing.

In regards to laser treatment, the presence of melasma in patients with darker skin tones makes post-inflammatory hyperpigmentation with any laser therapy a frequent complication. Melasma should be differentiated from post-inflammatory hyperpigmentation, which constitutes an inflammatory process. Once the causative factor is eliminated, then post-inflammatory hyperpigmentation is likely to resolve with treatment with a topical retinoid and hydroquinone.[60] In contrast, melasma often requires prolong therapy. Topical hydroquinone or kojic acid preparations alone or in combination with chemical peels have been the treatment of choice.[61] Giving a laser test dose at a minimally conspicuous location (ie, behind the auricle) should be considered to determine its future pigmentary response.

Managing Recurrent Keloids

For recurrent earlobe keloids with previous excision and steroid treatment, repeat surgical excision followed by radiation therapy within 1 week of excision is a possible option after careful discussion with the patient. For recurrent keloids at other head and neck regions, post-operative radiation is more controversial due to risk of radiation exposure to the salivary and thyroid glands. Following excision, silicone occlusive sheeting or gel over the site for 12 hours a day for 6 months is beneficial. On the earlobe, pressure clip on earrings can be applied.

The off-label use of topical mitomycin C or intralesional 5-fluorouracil can be considered for the treatment of recalcitrant keloids with proper patient consent.[62] The patient must be informed of the possibility of neoplastic transformation with this therapy.

Other miscellaneous pharmacologic therapies to treat keloids include topical retinoic acid, colchicine, antihistamines, lathyrogens, putrescine, zinc, vitamin A, vitamin E, verapamil, and interferons, whose efficacies are yet to be determined. In the future, a standardized grading system is needed to measure the volume and quality of keloids to allow for more objective treatment comparisons between treatment regimens.

STRATUM CORNEUM AND EPIDERMIS

Although the major target for scar therapy is the dermis, topically applied treatments are also used, particularly when the more superficial features require modification and/or when scar therapies result, for example, in hyper or hypopigmentation. The influence of inherent skin color on SC and epidermal structure and function is provided.

The literature on the effects of ethnicity on SC barrier integrity, measured as transepidermal water loss (TEWL), is variable. Two studies showed no differences in vivo for forearm skin in African American, Hispanic, and Caucasian subjects.[63,64] Another comparison showed greater barrier integrity (lower TEWL) for African American versus Caucasians.[65] However, body site differences were noted with greater integrity for the upper arm versus the forearm. Barrier integrity was greater for African Americans than East Asians and both groups had lower TEWL than Caucasians at sites on the face.[66] In another study, facial skin TEWL was lower in African American women than in age-matched Caucasians, indicating a more effective SC barrier.[67] Overall SC thickness did not differ for blacks versus whites.[64] The number of tape strippings required to compromise the facial SC barrier (typically defined as 2–3 times higher than baseline) differed significantly for all 3 groups with more strips in African Americans, indicating a stronger barrier, versus Caucasians and East Asians.[66]

SC lipid compositions were examined in cohorts of Caucasians, Asians, and Africans. The ceramide/cholesterol ratio was significantly lower in Africans versus Asians and Africans versus Caucasians but the 3 groups were comparable for the ceramide subgroups.[68] Facial skin samples from African subjects had lower amounts of ceramides compared with Caucasian and East Asian groups.[66] Skin surface lipids were compared with facial skin of African American, Northern Asian, and Caucasians. The amounts were greater in Africans, with the wax ester fraction and the distribution of 6 wax ester fatty acids differing for all 3 groups in the order African > Asian > Caucasian.[67]

Greater incidence of self-assessed skin sensitivity and a greater neurosensory response to topically applied agents, for example, lactic acid, acetic acid, and capsaicin, have been reported for Asians compared with Caucasians, although standard acute irritation tests produced similar findings.[69,70] Other factors, including the presence of a polymorphism at position-308 in the tumor necrosis factor α gene and an atopic diathesis, in addition to specific color and functional differences may account for the differences.[71,72] Nonetheless, sensitivity to topical agents is an important consideration for selection of treatment. Collectively, these findings suggest that additional studies will be needed to discern the cause of ethnic variation in SC structure and function.

REFERENCES

1. Peacock EE Jr, Madden JW, Trier WC. Biologic basis for the treatment of keloids and hypertrophic scars. South Med J 1970;63(7):755–60.
2. Parrett BM, Donelan MB. Pulsed dye laser in burn scars: current concepts and future directions. Burns 2010;36(4):443–9.
3. Serup J. Skin irritation: objective characterization in a clinical perspective. In: Wilhelm KP, Elsner P, Berardesca E, et al, editors. Bioengineering of the skin: skin surface imaging and analysis. Boca Raton (FL): CRC Press; 1997. p. 261–73.
4. Stephen ID, Coetzee V, Law Smith M, et al. Skin blood perfusion and oxygenation colour affect perceived human health. PLoS One 2009;4(4):e5083.
5. Galdino GM, Vogel JE, Vander Kolk CA. Standardizing digital photography: it's not all in the eye of the beholder. Plast Reconstr Surg 2001;108(5):1334–44.
6. Anderson RR, Parrish JA. The optics of human skin. J Invest Dermatol 1981;77(1):13–9.
7. Taylor S, Westerhof W, Im S, et al. Noninvasive techniques for the evaluation of skin color. J Am Acad Dermatol 2006;54(5 Suppl 2):S282–90.
8. Fink B, Matts PJ. The effects of skin colour distribution and topography cues on the perception of female facial age and health. J Eur Acad Dermatol Venereol 2008;22(4):493–8.
9. Fink B, Matts PJ, Klingenberg H, et al. Visual attention to variation in female facial skin color distribution. J Cosmet Dermatol 2008;7(2):155–61.
10. Fink B, Grammer K, Matts PJ. Visual skin color distribution plays a role in the perception of age, attractiveness, and health of female faces. Evol Hum Behav 2006;27(6):433–42.
11. Matts PJ, Fink B. Chronic sun damage and the perception of age, health and attractiveness. Photochem Photobiol Sci 2010;9(4):421–31.
12. Arce-Lopera C, Igarashi T, Nakao K, et al. Image statistics on the age perception of human skin. Skin Res Technol 2013;19(1):e273–8.
13. Chardon A, Cretois I, Hourseau C. Skin colour typology and suntanning pathways. Int J Cosmet Sci 1991;13(4):191–208.
14. Stamatas GN, Zmudzka BZ, Kollias N, et al. Non-invasive measurements of skin pigmentation in situ. Pigment Cell Res 2004;17(6):618–26.
15. Takiwaki H. Measurement of skin color: practical application and theoretical considerations. J Med Invest 1998;44(3–4):121–6.
16. Sullivan T, Smith J, Kermode J, et al. Rating the burn scar. J Burn Care Rehabil 1990;11(3):256–60.
17. Weller R, Hunter J, Savin J, et al. Cinical dermatology. 4th edition. Malden (MA): Blackwell Publishing; 2008.
18. von Luschan F. Beitrage zur Volkerkunde der Deutschen Schutzgebienen. Berlin: Deutsche Buchgemeinschaft; 1897.
19. Nordlund JJ, Boissy RE. The biology of melanocytes. In: Freinkel RK, Woodley DT, editors. The biology of the skin. New York: Parthenon Publishing Group; 2001. p. 113–31.
20. Alaluf S, Atkins D, Barrett K, et al. Ethnic variation in melanin content and composition in photoexposed and photoprotected human skin. Pigment Cell Res 2002;15(2):112–8.
21. Chan HH. Special considerations for darker-skinned patients. Curr Probl Dermatol 2011;42:153–9.
22. Morgan JE, Gilchrest B, Goldwyn RM. Skin pigmentation. Current concepts and relevance to plastic surgery. Plast Reconstr Surg 1975;56(6):617–28.
23. Knudsen A, Brodersen R. Skin colour and bilirubin in neonates. Arch Dis Child 1989;64(4):605–9.
24. Lock-Andersen J, Wulf HC. Seasonal variation of skin pigmentation. Acta Derm Venereol 1997;77(3):219–21.
25. Shriver MD, Parra EJ. Comparison of narrow-band reflectance spectroscopy and tristimulus colorimetry for measurements of skin and hair color in persons of different biological ancestry. Am J Phys Anthropol 2000;112(1):17–27.

26. Clarys P, Alewaeters K, Lambrecht R, et al. Skin color measurements: comparison between three instruments: the Chromameter(R), the DermaSpectrometer(R) and the Mexameter(R). Skin Res Technol 2000;6(4):230–8.

27. Girardeau-Hubert S, Pageon H, Asselineau D. In vivo and in vitro approaches in understanding the differences between Caucasian and African skin types: specific involvement of the papillary dermis. Int J Dermatol 2012;51(Suppl 1):1–4.

28. Berardesca E, Maibach H. Cutaneous reactive hyperaemia: racial differences induced by corticoid application. Br J Dermatol 1989;120(6):787–94.

29. Bayat A, McGrouther DA, Ferguson MW. Skin scarring. BMJ 2003;326(7380):88–92.

30. Gauglitz GG, Korting HC, Pavicic T, et al. Hypertrophic scarring and keloids: pathomechanisms and current and emerging treatment strategies. Mol Med 2011;17(1–2):113–25.

31. Kischer CW, Thies AC, Chvapil M. Perivascular myofibroblasts and microvascular occlusion in hypertrophic scars and keloids. Hum Pathol 1982;13(9):819–24.

32. Ehrlich HP, Desmouliere A, Diegelmann RF, et al. Morphological and immunochemical differences between keloid and hypertrophic scar. Am J Pathol 1994;145(1):105–13.

33. Lawrence JW, Mason ST, Schomer K, et al. Epidemiology and impact of scarring after burn injury: a systematic review of the literature. J Burn Care Res 2012;33(1):136–46.

34. Passaretti D, Billmire DA. Management of pediatric burns. J Craniofac Surg 2003;14(5):713–8.

35. Soltani AM, Francis CS, Motamed A, et al. Hypertrophic scarring in cleft lip repair: a comparison of incidence among ethnic groups. Clin Epidemiol 2012;4:187–91.

36. Ud-Din S, Bayat A. Strategic management of keloid disease in ethnic skin: a structured approach supported by the emerging literature. Br J Dermatol 2013;169(Suppl 3):71–81.

37. Santucci M, Borgognoni L, Reali UM, et al. Keloids and hypertrophic scars of Caucasians show distinctive morphologic and immunophenotypic profiles. Virchows Arch 2001;438(5):457–63.

38. Brown JJ, Ollier WE, Arscott G, et al. Association of HLA-DRB1* and keloid disease in an Afro-Caribbean population. Clin Exp Dermatol 2010;35(3):305–10.

39. de las Alas JM, Siripunvarapon AH, Dofitas BL. Pulsed dye laser for the treatment of keloid and hypertrophic scars: a systematic review. Expert Rev Med Devices 2012;9(6):641–50.

40. Hom D. Treating the elusive Keloid. Arch Otolaryngol Head Neck Surg 2001;127:1140–3.

41. Draaijers LJ, Tempelman FR, Botman YA, et al. Colour evaluation in scars: tristimulus colorimeter, narrow-band simple reflectance meter or subjective evaluation? Burns 2004;30(2):103–7.

42. Nedelec B, Shankowsky HA, Tredget EE. Rating the resolving hypertrophic scar: comparison of the Vancouver Scar Scale and scar volume. J Burn Care Rehabil 2000;21(3):205–12.

43. Sproat JE, Dalcin A, Weitauer N, et al. Hypertrophic sternal scars: silicone gel sheet versus Kenalog injection treatment. Plast Reconstr Surg 1992;90(6):988–92.

44. Janssen de Limpens AM. The local treatment of hypertrophic scars and keloids with topical retinoic acid. Br J Dermatol 1980;103(3):319–23.

45. Fulton JE Jr. Silicone gel sheeting for the prevention and management of evolving hypertrophic and keloid scars. Dermatol Surg 1995;21(11):947–51.

46. Musgrave MA, Umraw N, Fish JS, et al. The effect of silicone gel sheets on perfusion of hypertrophic burn scars. J Burn Care Rehabil 2002;23(3):208–14.

47. Chang P, Laubenthal KN, Lewis RW 2nd, et al. Prospective, randomized study of the efficacy of pressure garment therapy in patients with burns. J Burn Care Rehabil 1995;16(5):473–5.

48. Patino O, Novick C, Merlo A, et al. Massage in hypertrophic scars. J Burn Care Rehabil 1999;20(3):268–71 [discussion: 267].

49. Clayton JL, Edkins R, Cairns BA, et al. Incidence and management of adverse events after the use of laser therapies for the treatment of hypertrophic burn scars. Ann Plast Surg 2013;70(5):500–5.

50. Hultman CS, Edkins RE, Lee CN, et al. Shine on: review of laser- and light-based therapies for the treatment of burn scars. Dermatol Res Pract 2012;2012:243651.

51. Bailey JK, Burkes SA, Visscher MO, et al. Multimodal quantitative analysis of early pulsed-dye laser treatment of scars at a pediatric burn hospital. Dermatol Surg 2012;38(9):1490–6.

52. Nouri K, Jimenez GP, Harrison-Balestra C, et al. 585-nm pulsed dye laser in the treatment of surgical scars starting on the suture removal day. Dermatol Surg 2003;29(1):65–73 [discussion: 73].

53. Battle EF Jr, Soden CE Jr. The use of lasers in darker skin types. Semin Cutan Med Surg 2009;28(2):130–40.

54. Anderson RR. Laser-tissue interactions in dermatology. Philadelphia: Lippincott-Raven; 1997.

55. Manuskiatti W, Eimpunth S, Wanitphakdeedecha R. Effect of cold air cooling on the incidence of postinflammatory hyperpigmentation after Q-switched Nd:YAG laser treatment of acquired bilateral nevus of Ota like macules. Arch Dermatol 2007;143(9):1139–43.

56. Tanzi EL, Alster TS. Comparison of a 1450-nm diode laser and a 1320-nm Nd:YAG laser in the

treatment of atrophic facial scars: a prospective clinical and histologic study. Dermatol Surg 2004; 30(2 Pt 1):152–7.

57. Chan NP, Ho SG, Yeung CK, et al. The use of non-ablative fractional resurfacing in Asian acne scar patients. Lasers Surg Med 2010;42(10):710–5.

58. Lindsey W, Davis P. Facial keloids. A 15-year experience. Arch Otolaryngol Head Neck Surg 1997; 123:397–400.

59. Rusciani L, Rossi G, Bono R. Use of cryotherapy in the treatment of keloids. J Dermatol Surg Oncol 1993;19:529–34.

60. Callender VD. Considerations for treating acne in ethnic skin. Cutis 2005;76(Suppl 2):19–23.

61. Jackson BA. Lasers in ethnic skin: a review. J Am Acad Dermatol 2003;48(Suppl 6):S134–8.

62. Stewart CE 4th, Kim JY. Application of mitomycin-C for head and neck keloids. Otolaryngol Head Neck Surg 2006;135(6):946–50.

63. Berardesca E, de Rigal J, Leveque JL, et al. In vivo biophysical characterization of skin physiological differences in races. Dermatologica 1991;182(2):89–93.

64. Berardesca E, Maibach H. Ethnic skin: overview of structure and function. J Am Acad Dermatol 2003; 48(Suppl 6):S139–42.

65. Chu M, Kollias N. Documentation of normal stratum corneum scaling in an average population: features of differences among age, ethnicity and body site. Br J Dermatol 2011;164(3):497–507.

66. Muizzuddin N, Hellemans L, Van Overloop L, et al. Structural and functional differences in barrier properties of African American, Caucasian and East Asian skin. J Dermatol Sci 2010;59(2):123–8.

67. Pappas A, Fantasia J, Chen T. Age and ethnic variations in sebaceous lipids. Dermatoendocrinol 2013;5(2):319–24.

68. Jungersted JM, Hogh JK, Hellgren LI, et al. Ethnicity and stratum corneum ceramides. Br J Dermatol 2010;163(6):1169–73.

69. Lee E, Kim S, Lee J, et al. Ethnic differences in objective and subjective skin irritation response: an international study. Skin Res Technol 2013. [Epub ahead of print].

70. Robinson MK. Racial differences in acute and cumulative skin irritation responses between Caucasian and Asian populations. Contact Dermatitis 2000;42(3):134–43.

71. Davis JA, Visscher MO, Wickett RR, et al. Influence of tumour necrosis factor-alpha polymorphism-308 and atopy on irritant contact dermatitis in healthcare workers. Contact Dermatitis 2010;63(6):320–32.

72. Davis JA, Visscher MO, Wickett RR, et al. Role of TNF-alpha polymorphism -308 in neurosensory irritation. Int J Cosmet Sci 2011;33(2):105–12.

Considerations in Non-Caucasian Facial Rejuvenation

Jonathan M. Sykes, MD*, David Nolen, MD

KEYWORDS

- Facelift • Rhytidectomy • Genioplasty • Chin augmentation

KEY POINTS

- Ethnic facial characterizations have been described in the literature but have become more blended in modern society.
- It is important to understand facial skeletal variations and how that affects soft tissue support, facial features, and facial aging.
- Pigmented skin has larger fibroblasts and higher lipid content than lighter skin; this, along with increased dermal thickening, affects the manner of aging of the face and healing after rejuvenative procedures.
- Deep plane rhytidectomy should be considered over a mini-lift and superficial rhytidectomy in many Asian patients.
- Chin augmentation can be a beneficial procedure in Asian patients with a less projected bony pogonion who seek facial rejuvenation.

INTRODUCTION

Aging of the face is inevitable and undeniable. Facial aging includes a loss of skeletal support, soft tissue volume depletion, and a decrease in skin elasticity. Surgical rejuvenation of the face includes a variety of procedures designed to restore soft tissue volume, reestablish skeletal support, and reposition ptotic soft tissues.

To rejuvenate any face, the facial plastic surgeon must diagnose the specific cause of the aging process, requiring attention to the anatomic causes of the individual's aging. Each face is individual in its rate and specific type of aging. Although every face is unique, certain facial types exist that loosely dictate how that face will age. This article outlines the pertinent anatomy related to facial aging and the characteristics of certain facial types and ethnicities and presents an algorithm for treatment of each aging types.

ANATOMIC CONSIDERATIONS OF FACIAL AGING

The anatomic layers of the face are consistent in all faces. These layers, from superficial to deep, are the skin, subcutaneous fat, superficial fascia, loose areolar tissue, and deep fascia. Although the layers in all faces are the same, the relative thicknesses and the tendency to slide on each other are variable. It is clear that the amount of fat varies in each face according to face type, genetics, body mass index (BMI), and ethnicity.[1] Each of these characteristics contributes to the overall amount of facial volume and to the manner that the face ages.

The pathophysiology of facial aging includes (1) loss of skin elasticity, (2) soft tissue volume depletion, and (3) loss of skeletal support of the soft tissue envelope.[2] Surgical rejuvenation of the face should be individualized to reestablish skeletal

Disclosures: None.
Facial Plastic and Reconstructive Surgery, UC Davis Medical Center, 2521 Stockton Boulevard, Suite 6206, Sacramento, CA 95746, USA
* Corresponding author.
E-mail address: jonathan.sykes@ucdmc.ucdavis.edu

Facial Plast Surg Clin N Am 22 (2014) 463–470
http://dx.doi.org/10.1016/j.fsc.2014.04.008
1064-7406/14/$ – see front matter © 2014 Elsevier Inc. All rights reserved.

support and/or replenish soft tissue volume loss and to lift soft tissues when they are ptotic.

Mitz and Peyronie[3] provided the original description (1976) of the superficial fascia of the face, the superficial musculoaponeurotic system (SMAS). This fascia envelopes the midface and interconnects the midfacial musculature. In all areas of the head and neck (the forehead, temple, midface, and neck), the superficial fascia connects to the deep fascia through fibrous interconnections (loose areolar tissue). The density of this loose areolar tissue is quite variable and determines the amount that the soft tissues of the face sag. The superficial to deep fascial attachment can be dense or consist of loose filmy tissue that slides easily on each other.

In thin patients with low BMI, there is relatively less subcutaneous fat and the glide plane between the superficial and deep fascia is characterized by a loose attachment. This weak attachment leads to a lack of support and ptosis of the soft tissues. In patients with denser facial fat, the thicker subcutaneous layer is usually associated with less facial rhytids and less descent of the soft tissues of the face.

ANATOMIC CHARACTERISTICS OF DIFFERENT RACES

There is no standard facial type for any race or ethnicity. As societies have changed, a mingling of facial characteristics of Asian, Caucasian, and Negroid features has occurred. This cross-fertilization has blurred facial characteristic and classic distinctions between races.

In the past, it was common to hear lectures or read articles in the plastic surgery literature highlighting the specific facial characteristics of a particular race or ethnicity. Presently, it is not accurate to characterize a facial type based on ethnicity, as there is no Mestizo nose, or Asian facial type.

However, it is clear that certain faces have denser and more globular fat, and this causes aging that is different than those individuals who lose fat and facial volume as they age. The tendencies to lose versus maintain fat as one ages depends on several factors, including body weight and the individual's particular genetic composition. For instance, if a patient's parents tend toward good maintenance of facial volume (as they aged), the chances are high that that individual will maintain his or her facial volume as they age.

The characteristic facial skeleton in most Asian patients is a prominent zygomaticomalar region with a large bizygomatic width.[4] The lower facial skeleton is often characterized by a less projected bony pogonion (weak chin) in the anterior-posterior direction.[5] However, the transverse width of the mandible (from one mandibular angle to the other) is usually large. This relatively masculine trait often causes women to request bony mandibular angle reduction.[6] The dental skeletal relation in Asian patients often reveals bimaxillary protrusion. Bimaxillary protrusion is associated with a weak position of the bony subnasale and a weak pogonion, but a prominent dental occlusion in the anterior-posterior dimension.[7] For this reason, chin augmentation with either an alloplast chin implant or a horizontal osteotomy of the bony mentum (sliding bony genioplasty) is a complementary procedure to lifting in lower facial rejuvenation.[8] In that bimaxillary protrusion is associated with a slightly protuberant lower lip, the lower lip should not be used solely as a reference point when deciding on the size of the chin implant and the desired amount of augmentation. Conservative augmentation of the chin should be performed in a balancing procedure (Figs. 1 and 2).

SKIN CONSIDERATIONS

In most Asian patients, the skin is thicker and more fibrous than is skin in Caucasians.[9] In addition, there is more pigment and tendency for solar lentigines. The effects of thicker skin with increased pigmentation are important for the patient desiring facial rejuvenation.[5] On average, skin in Asian patients has increased dermal thickness, collagen content, and melanin than skin in Caucasians. Studies comparing racial differences in the structure of the stratum corneum suggest that more pigmented skin contains more cell layers when compared with lightly pigmented skin. Pigmented skin also has larger fibroblasts and higher lipid content than lighter skin.[10,11]

The larger fibroblasts and increased dermal thickening in Asians affect both the manner of aging of the face and the healing after rejuvenative procedures.[12] In 2005, Nouveau-Richard and colleagues[13] studied aging characteristics in age-matched populations of Chinese and Europeans. This study revealed that the onset of wrinkles in Asian women was delayed by approximately 10 years when compared with age-matched French women. In addition, aging Asian women had an increased association of noncancerous pigmented lesions when compared with European women.

PROCEDURE SELECTION

The skin type of Asian patients not only results in less wrinkles and increased pigmented lesions

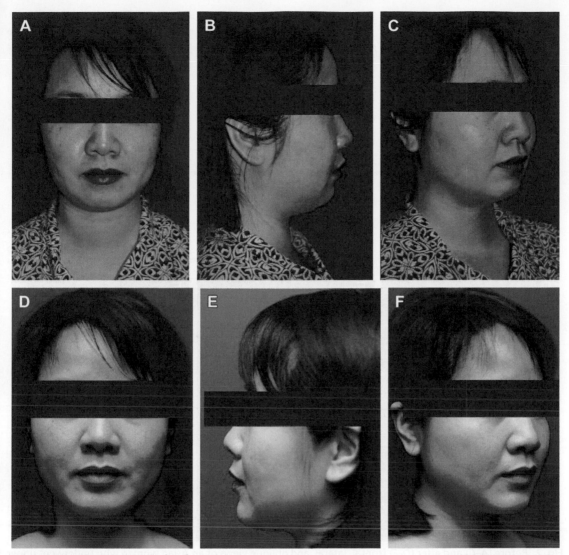

Fig. 1. (*A–C*) Before and (*D–F*) after frontal, lateral, and oblique views of an Asian woman who underwent a chin implant, submental liposuction, and neck lift.

with aging, but also affects the healing process when aging procedures are performed. Increased dermal thickness results in a higher incidence of hypertrophic scars in Asian patients,[14] which may increase the chance of having an unfavorable scar after procedures such as rhytidectomy or blepharoplasty. In addition, scarring after nonsurgical procedures, such as skin resurfacing or laser treatment of cutaneous lesions, may be adversely affected.

It is important that the surgeon understands the patient's motivations for, and expectations of, plastic surgery. The options for therapy, as well as the expected results and limitations of any procedure or procedures, should be discussed. Some

requests may be cultural (for example, the desire to surgically narrow a wide bigonial angle). Some requests may reflect the aging process (for example, the wish for less resurfacing procedures and more procedures to lessen pigmented lesions). In any case, clear communication accounting for the patient's wishes and discussing the expected outcomes of therapy is essential to achieve patient satisfaction.

The surgical procedures commonly used to rejuvenate the aging face in Asians include lifting and support of the deep fascial structures of the midface and lower face.[15] Because the superficial fat and soft tissues are often dense in Asians, minimal lifting procedures such as mini-lifts or cable lifts

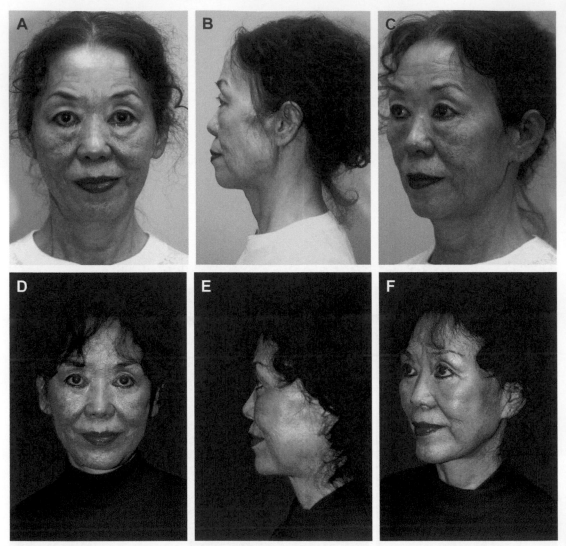

Fig. 2. Before (*A–C*) and after (*D–F*) frontal, lateral, and oblique views of an Asian woman who underwent upper and lower blepharoplasty, deep plane rhytidectomy with submental liposuction, platysmaplasty, and chin augmentation with alloplastic implant.

usually are inadequate to provide necessary support to provide long-term facial rejuvenation. Cable lifts have the advantage of limited cutaneous incisions and minimal postsurgical downtime. However, the lack of complete separation of tissue planes associated with these procedures usually does not overcome the gravitational forces that result postoperatively. Mini-lifts performed in a plane superficial to the SMAS are also usually inadequate, as these procedures also do not provide necessary structural lifting.

DEEP PLANE RHYTIDECTOMY

The deep plane facelift allows for maximum tension on the deep structures and is the procedure

chosen by the senior author for midfacial and lower facial lifting (**Fig. 3**). This technique involves creating a facelift flap with minimal subcutaneous elevation in the preauricular region. Most of the flap is then elevated in the sub-SMAS dissection plane. The thicker flap allows for maximal tension on the deep tissues and vertical vector elevation of the soft tissues of the face. In theory, increased tension on the deep tissues with less tension on the skin flap allows for improved cutaneous scarring (vs the scars that would result from a subcutaneous flap elevation).

Originally described by Hamra,[16] the deep plane facelift transitions from the subcutaneous plane in the immediate preauricular region to the sub-SMAS plane at a line between the mandibular

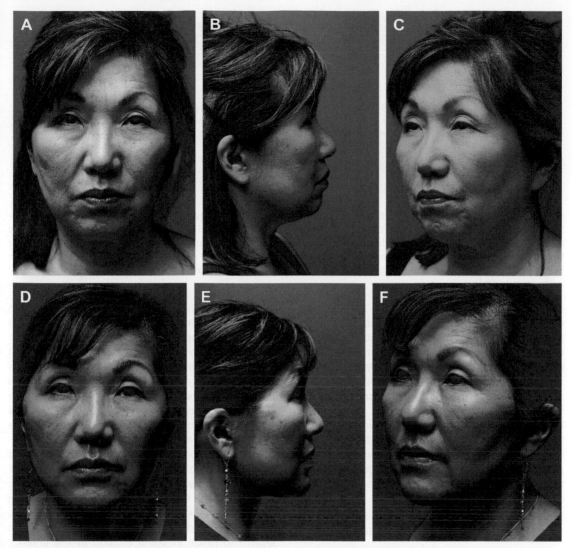

Fig. 3. (*A–F*) Before and after frontal, lateral, and oblique views of an Asian woman who underwent a deep plane rhytidectomy. Superficial lifts would be inadequate to achieve the goals of this patient.

angle and the lateral canthus. Dissecting deep to the SMAS anterior to this described artificial line allows for safe elevation and mobilization of the SMAS (**Fig. 4**). The technique involves complete division of the mandibulocutaneous and zygomaticocutaneous ligaments.[16] After full release of the facial soft tissues, the facelift flap is fixated to the deep temporal fascia with monofilament long-acting absorbable sutures. Vertical flap elevation allows improvement in both the midfacial and the cervical soft tissues.

TREATMENT OF THE NECK

The approach and treatment of the neck are variable according to the patient's specific anatomy.

The goal of neck surgery is to improve neck contour and to decrease the cervicomental angle. In patients with limited laxity of the neck soft tissues, the anterior neck is not opened and improvement is obtained with a lateral pull on the free edge of the platysma muscle to the mastoid periosteum. In patients with a small amount of submental fat excess, a small incision is used and only submental liposuction or direct excision is performed. In these cases, it is important to leave an adequate amount of fat on the submental flap and not to remove too much submental fat; this will avoid contour abnormalities of the skin and the "cobra-neck" deformity.

If the patient has more skin and/or fat excess, a longer (2–3 cm) incision may be necessary to

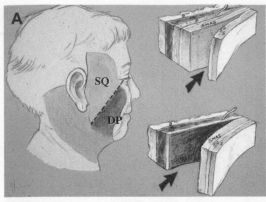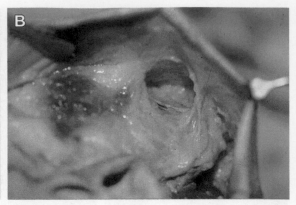

Fig. 4. (*A*) The flap transitions from the subcutaneous plane (SQ) in the immediate preauricular region to the sub-SMAS plane (DP) at a line between the mandibular angle and the lateral canthus. The top *arrow* points to the superficial plane of dissection, and the bottom *arrow* points to the deep plane of dissection that occurs anterior to the drawn line. (*B*) Transition between the subcutaneous plane and the deep plane in a cadaveric study. (*From* Sykes JM. Management of the aging face in the Asian patient. Facial Plast Surg Clin North Am 2007;15(3):356; with permission.)

contour and redrape the neck soft tissues adequately. In these cases, direct excision of sub-platysmal fat is often required for neck contour. A small amount of platysma muscle (medial margin) resection is usually also necessary for desired soft tissue recontouring. After removal of fat and medial platysma muscle, suturing of the medial free edges of the platysma muscle is necessary to tighten the central sling and to avoid any soft tissue contour irregularities (**Fig. 5**). In cases of significant central submental excess, resection of a portion of the anterior belly of the digastric muscle with central corset plication of this muscle enhances cervical definition.

SKELETAL ENHANCEMENT—GENIOPLASTY

The selection of the best procedure to correct a given deformity of the chin should be based on the type and extent of the deformity. Augmentation of the chin with an alloplastic implant is a simple and effective method of correcting a horizontal chin deficiency. This technique is limited by the availability of various sizes and shapes of alloplastic implants. Chin augmentation with implants is also less effective in patients with significant vertical discrepancies (vertical excess or deficiency). Placement of an implant in such a patient may exacerbate the vertical excess and make the chin appear longer. For these reasons, implant augmentation is an effective method of camouflage for minor chin deformities, but may not be satisfactory for complex deformities.

It is very common for Asian patients to exhibit bimaxillary protrusion and microgenia.[2,7] In these patients, the dental arches are anterior and the chin is horizontally deficient. It is important to augment the chin conservatively in patients with this condition, as overaugmentation can produce an unnatural appearance.

Either an intraoral or an external (submental) incision and approach can be used to place a chin implant. If an extraoral approach is used, an incision (approximately 2–3 cm) is made in the submental crease and carried through the dermis and subcutaneous fat. The mentalis muscles are then divided to enter a dissection plane just superficial to the periosteum of the anterior face of the mandible. The chin implant can be placed in either the subperiosteal or the supraperiosteal plane. The advantage of placing an implant beneath the periosteum is improved fixation of the implant. However, subperiosteal placement has been shown to result in some erosion of the anterior mandible. For these reasons, most surgeons advocate dissection in the supraperiosteal plane centrally, with subperiosteal placement laterally, theoretically minimizing mandibular erosion, while maximally fixing the implant.

Osteotomy of the bony mentum (osseous genioplasty) is a versatile and reliable procedure for correcting a variety of skeletal chin deformities. First described by Hofer in 1942,[17] this technique involves horizontal osteotomy and downfracture of the chin, with repositioning and fixation of the distal segment. Osseous genioplasty allows advancement or retrusion in the AP direction, as well as lengthening or shortening in the vertical direction.[8] In addition, the genioplasty procedure provides an approach for correction of transverse asymmetries of the chin. In patients with significant asymmetry of the lower third, or with significant vertical deficiency or excess, bony genioplasty is the preferred treatment for microgenia (**Fig. 6**).

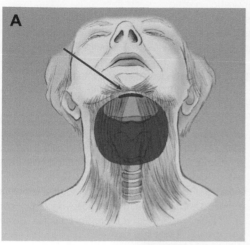

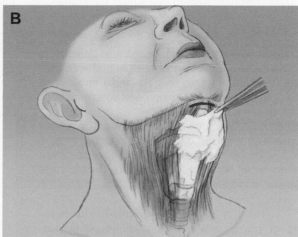

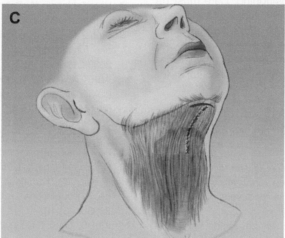

Fig. 5. (*A*) Placement of a submental incision that is made in patients that need submental liposuction. The extent of dissection depends on the patient's needs and amount of submental fat. The lightly shaded region depicts what is needed in a patient with only a small amount of excess submental fat, and the darker shading indicates a more extensive area of fat resection that is needed in a heavy neck. (*B*) In a patient with a full, heavy neck, fat resection is performed in a supra-subplatysmal. Leaving the subplatysmal fat can lead to compromised results in the contour of the neck. (*C*) Corsett platysmaplasty is performed in patients that have anterior platysmal banding or in patients that have required more extensive fat resection to avoid contour deformities. (*From* Sykes JM. Management of the aging face in the Asian patient. Facial Plast Surg Clin North Am 2007;15(3):358; with permission.)

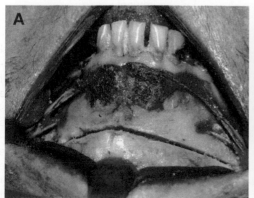

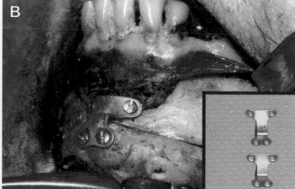

Fig. 6. (*A*) Cadaveric dissection showing the placement of the osteotomy below the level of the mental foramina. (*B*) Stair step plates are used to fix the osteotomy in place and prevent movement during the healing phase.

SUMMARY

Rejuvenation of the aged face requires attention to a variety of anatomic and aesthetic characteristics. The facial plastic surgeon must understand the specific variations in skin and soft tissues, as well as in skeletal architecture.

Although faces can and should never be stereotyped, characteristics of Asian faces include thicker skin with a tendency for increased pigmentation when scarring. In addition, Asians have denser subcutaneous fat with less cutaneous rhytids.

Treatment of aging faces in Asians requires lifting of ptotic soft tissues often requiring sub-SMAS elevation and repositioning. Care must be taken to avoid excess wound tension to minimize cutaneous scarring. Most importantly, good communication with patients should involve discussing the goals and limitations of any procedures and setting reasonable expectations for surgical results.

REFERENCES

1. Wan D, Amirlak B, Giessler P. The differing adipocyte morphologies of deep versus superficial midfacial fat compartments: a cadaveric study. Plast Reconstr Surg 2014;133(5):615e–22e.
2. Sykes JM. Management of the aging face in the Asian patient. Facial Plast Surg Clin North Am 2007;15(3):353–60.
3. Mitz V, Peyronie M. The superficial musculoapaneurotic system (SMAS) in the parotoid and cheek area. Plast Reconstr Surg 1976;58:80–8.
4. Guo MK. Cephalometric standards of Steiner analysis established on Chinese children. Taiwan Yi Xue Hui Za Zhi 1971;70(2):97–102.
5. Shirakabe Y, Suzuki Y, Lam S. A new paradigm for the aging Asian face. Aesthetic Plast Surg 2003; 27(5):397–402.
6. Li J, Hsu Y, Khadka A, et al. Contouring of a square jaw on a short face by narrowing and sliding genioplasty combined with mandibular outer cortex ostectomy in orientals. Plast Reconstr Surg 2011;127(5): 2083–92.
7. Chu YM, Bergeron L, Chen YR. Bimaxillary protrusion: an overview of the surgical-orthodontic treatment. Semin Plast Surg 2009;23(1):32–9.
8. Sykes S, Frodel J. Mentoplasty and facial implants. In: Flint C, editor. Cummings Otolaryngology Head and Neck Surgery. 5th edition. Philadelphia: Elsevier; 2010. p. 461–74.
9. Lee Y, Hwang K. Skin thickness of Korean adults. Surg Radiol Anat 2002;24(3–4):183–9.
10. Richards GM, Oresajo CO, Halder RM. Structure and function of ethnic skin and hair. Dermatol Clin 2003;21(4):595–600.
11. Abe T, Arai S, Mimura K, et al. Studies of physiological factors affecting skin susceptibility to ultraviolet light irradiation and irritants. J Dermatol 1983; 10(6):531–7.
12. Yu SS, Grekin RC. Aesthetic analysis of Asian skin. Facial Plast Surg Clin North Am 2007;15(3):361–5,. vii.
13. Nouveau-Richard S, Yang Z, Mac-Mary S, et al. Skin ageing: a comparison between Chinese and European populations. A pilot study. J Dermatol Sci 2005;40(3):187–93.
14. Kim S, Choi TH, Liu W. Update on scar management: guidelines for treating Asian patients. Plast Reconstr Surg 2013;132(6):1580–9.
15. Bergeron L, Chen YR. The Asian face lift. Semin Plast Surg 2009;23(1):40–7.
16. Hamra ST. The deep-plane rhytidectomy. Plast Reconstr Surg 1990;86(1):53–61.
17. Hofer O. Operation der prognathie und mikrogenie. Deutsche Zahnarztl Mund Kief 1942;9:121.

Index

Note: Page numbers of article titles are in **boldface** type.

Facial Plast Surg Clin N Am 22 (2014) 471–486
http://dx.doi.org/10.1016/S1064-7406(14)00068-6
1064-7406/14/$ – see front matter © 2014 Elsevier Inc. All rights reserved.

Printed and bound by CPI Group (UK) Ltd, Croydon, CR0 4YY

03/10/2024

01040375-0012